THE
DIABETES
SOURCEBOOK

Fifth Edition

Diana W. Guthrie, Ph.D., A.R.N.P., and Richard A. Guthrie, M.D.
Certified Diabetes Educators

McGraw-Hill

New York   Chicago   San Francisco   Lisbon   London   Madrid   Mexico City
Milan   New Delhi   San Juan   Seoul   Singapore   Sydney   Toronto

Library of Congress Cataloging-in-Publication Data

Guthrie, Diana W.
    The diabetes sourcebook / by Diana W. Guthrie and Richard A. Guthrie ; foreword
by June Biermann and Barbara Toohey. — 5th ed.
       p.   cm.
    Includes bibliographical references and index.
    ISBN 0-7373-0642-4 (alk. paper)
    1. Diabetes—Popular works.   I. Guthrie, Richard A., 1935–   II. Title.

RC660.4 .G88   2003
616.4'62—dc21   2003048500

*This book is dedicated to our family
for the sacrifices they made so that we would
have time to write this book, and to
June Biermann and Barbara Toohey for the
tremendous contributions they have made
to people who have diabetes.*

2 3 4 5 6 7 8 9 0   DOC/DOC   0 9 8 7 6 5 4 3

ISBN 0-7373-0642-4

8-20-04

Interior illustrations by Randy Miyake

McGraw-Hill books are available at special quantity discounts to use as premiums and sales
promotions, or for use in corporate training programs. For more information, please write to the
Director of Special Sales, Professional Publishing, McGraw-Hill, Two Penn Plaza, New York, NY
10121-2298. Or contact your local bookstore.

This book is printed on acid-free paper.

Contents

Foreword   vii
Acknowledgments   ix
Introduction   xi

1 What Kind of Diabetes Do You Have?   1

A Bit of History   1
Types of Diabetes   3
Problems Associated with Diabetes   8

2 Who Gets This Disease?   11

Early Forms of Diabetes   13
Gestational Diabetes   13
Secondary Types of Diabetes   14
Type 1 and Type 2 Diabetes   14

3 How Is Diabetes Treated?   21

Differences in Treatment for Children and Adults   21
Acute Care   25
Management of Type 1 Diabetes   26
Management of Type 2 Diabetes   29
Special Management Needs   30

4 What About Education?   33

Levels of Education   33
Choosing an Education Program   36
How Can Education Help You?   37

5   **How Should You Eat?**   39

Basic Eating Guidelines   40
Baseline Meal Planning   43
Special Needs   47

6   **What About Medications?**   51

Oral Diabetes Agents   52
Insulin   59
Methods of Insulin Delivery   66

7   **What Is Important About Exercise?**   77

Benefits of Exercise   77
Precautions in Exercising   80
The "Exercise Prescription"   83

8   **What About Hygiene?**   85

Dental Care   85
Skin Care   86
Foot Care   87
Eye Care   90
Sexually Related Hygiene   91

9   **How Is Diabetes Monitored?**   95

Frequency of Testing   96
What to Test   97
Management Approaches   100
Testing Supplies and Equipment   104
Summary   111

10   **What Are the Possible Complications of Diabetes?**   113

Acute Complications   114
Intermediate Complications   118
Chronic Complications   121
General information   130

11   **How Do You Adjust to Having Diabetes?**   133

Reacting to the Diagnosis   133
Family Support   137

12 How Does Stress Affect Diabetes?   **139**

   Acute Response   139
   Chronic Response   140
   Other Responses   141
   Stress Management   142

13 How Can You Help Your
Health Care Team Help You?   **149**

   Program Management   149
   Record Keeping   150

14 How Can You Help Your
Family and Friends Help You?   **155**

   Increasing Their Understanding   155
   Gaining Their Support   156
   Grieving   157
   Complementary and Alternative Choices   158

15 What Is Being Done to Conquer
Diabetes and Improve Its Management?   **159**

   Transplants   159
   Artificial Pancreas Transplants   162
   New Treatments   164
   Finding the Cause   168
   Update for Management of Type 1 and Type 2 Diabetes 170
   Funding for Research   172

Appendices   **175**

   Appendix A: Food Questionnaire   175
   Appendix B: Recommended Dietary Intakes   181
   Appendix C: American Diabetes Association
     Exchange Lists   187
   Appendix D: Meal Planning—Points in Nutrition   215
   Appendix E: Restaurant Guide Food Choices   219
   Appendix F: Metabolic (MET) Levels of Activities   227
   Appendix G: Some Activity and
     Exercise Caloric Expenditures   231

Appendix H: Resources   235
Appendix I: American Diabetes Association
    Division and Area Offices   239
Appendix J: Summer Camps for Children with Diabetes   243
Appendix K: Glossary of Diabetes-Related Terms   255
Appendix L: Diabetes-Related Websites   273

Bibliography   277

Index   283

Foreword

We first met Diana Guthrie back in 1979, when we were all nominated for the Ames Award as Outstanding Diabetes Educator of the Year. Diana won. As we became better acquainted with her and her endocrinologist husband, Richard, we quickly understood why. The Guthries, in their Wichita diabetes practice and their teaching at the University of Kansas School of Medicine at Wichita, have always been in the forefront of diabetes therapy and education and have generously given of themselves and their time to patients and colleagues.

We were often recipients of that generosity. When we wrote our *Diabetic's Total Health Book* and were advocating the then controversial relaxation therapies for stress reduction to lower blood sugars, we were able to draw heavily on the creative and innovative work done by the Guthries, work that vividly demonstrated the benefits of these therapies for diabetics and brought them into the realm of acceptance that they enjoy today.

Whenever we write a book on diabetes or our newsletter for diabetics, the *Health-O-Gram*, we continually rely on the Guthries for advice and counsel and fact checking. They have never let us and our readers down.

To give you an idea of the measure of respect the Guthries enjoy, once at an American Diabetes Association Annual Scientific Meeting, we were distributing complimentary copies of our *Diabetic's Total Health Book*, for which Diana had written the foreword. A large, formidable, and grouchy-looking woman, whose badge indicated that she was a diabetes nurse-educator, loomed before our table. "What's going on here?" she demanded.

"We're giving away copies of our new book."

She picked up a copy and looked it over with a jaundiced eye.

"It's free," we chorused brightly.

She still looked skeptical. Then her eye fell on Diana's name on the cover. "Well, if Diana Guthrie had something to do with it, it must be all right. I'll take one." With that she thrust the book into her tote bag and strode off.

And then not long ago we were talking to one of the country's leading endocrinologists—a former president of the American Association of Diabetes Educators. He had just relocated his practice from South Dakota to Kansas City. When we asked him why the move, he said, "I wanted to be closer to the Source."

"The Source?"

"Yes, the Diabetes Source, you know, the Guthries in Wichita."

This book will bring you to the Source, to the Guthries and all their knowledge, experience, and empathy. Drink freely here of the waters of health and life.

JUNE BIERMANN
BARBARA TOOHEY

Acknowledgments

Many people have contributed to this book, both directly and indirectly. Our mentor, Dr. Robert Jackson, has given us the appreciation of what we as professionals can learn from those who have the disease and from their family members. Our diabetes team—Deborah Hinnen, Lindy Childs, Judy Friesen, Kirby Conley, Karon Giles, Diana Rhiley, Jayne McDaniels, Mary Muncrief, Terry Burlakoff, Alicia Buckley, Marvel Logan, Julie Jamison, and Diane Mann—have contributed ideas, thoughts, and examples that were appropriate to the information presented on these pages. Their special areas of expertise have helped to make this book the resource that it is.

Special thanks go to Sharon Buller for her secretarial work. Special thanks go, too, to our children and grandchildren, who continually stimulate us to learn even more.

Someday, diabetes will be curable or, at least, preventable. Until then, it can be controlled. We trust that this book will aid those with the disease in controlling it, while living lives whose quality is enhanced by self-care practices.

Introduction

Diabetes mellitus is a disease (or, more properly, a syndrome or group of diseases) that is being diagnosed with increasing frequency. There are currently about 17 million people with diabetes in the United States. What's more, any child born in 2000 or after has a one in three chance of getting diabetes.

Although diabetes has been known for many, many years, its cause, its total impact on the body, and its genetic association still remain unsolved mysteries. Some of these mysteries are partially being revealed, but even as one door opens to the researcher, yet another door needs to be opened to find another answer.

There are varying theories as to what diabetes is and how it affects the body, and there are also various approaches to treating the disease. When a person is diagnosed as having this syndrome, the diagnosis affects not only that person but the rest of the family as well. Information is essential, both for understanding the disease and for preventing misconceptions. Therefore, ongoing education should be a significant part of any treatment program. This edition of *The Diabetes Sourcebook* presents updated information on self-care and includes some of the latest research. Perhaps even more important are the suggestions for how to work with health professionals.

This book is meant to be a resource for people who have diabetes and for their family members. It is not intended to give all the answers but to serve as a guide to further reading and resources. Health care professionals may also find this book useful as a tool for reviewing or increasing their education about the disease and its care. This book is intended not to replace classroom learning but to serve as a resource once that classroom information has been obtained. Supporting and teaching one another aids in the development of a good attitude about self-care, as does recognizing that there are many others in the same situation.

Good Diabetes Management

The control of diabetes to prevent or delay complications is more possible today than ever before. Education is a major key to seeking out those professionals who can provide quality education and care in order to attain high degrees of control. Since health professionals cannot live with the person or family twenty-four hours a day, seven days a week, self-management education is a must for anyone who is capable of learning such a process. Day-to-day changes or weekly changes aid in attaining the normalization of blood-glucose levels on a more frequent basis.

Most people can learn that it is possible for them to maintain normal blood-glucose levels for a sustained period of time (i.e., without the occurrence of any significant insulin reactions—below normal blood-glucose levels). The frustration comes for the individual who does "everything the doctor says" and still has problems with diabetes management.

We now recognize that there are types of insulin-dependent diabetes that are much more difficult to manage. But even individuals with these types of diabetes can learn to alter their food and medication in relation to their activities or emotional responses so that their bodies are able to mimic the nondiabetic state for longer periods of time. To do this, emotional support through family, community, and professionals is required. Management support through education and program prescription individualized for each person is needed.

About This Book

The Diabetes Sourcebook was written to assist in meeting these needs. This book is intended to guide a person's thinking in relation to the most frequently asked questions about the disease and its management. Its purpose is to guide the person or family to seek the medical assistance needed in order to conquer the potentially devastating effects of the disease before they occur.

This book starts off with the questions concerning what diabetes is and who gets it. Some guidance as to what should be known about the disease follows. We continue with how to treat diabetes, along with details concerning the components of this treatment, such as meal planning, medication, and exercise. Yes, there are problems. These are dealt with next. These problems include those that are acute, occurring along the way, and those that are termed "chronic complications." It then follows that if you have diabetes, know about the disease, and treat it, you will be able to monitor it so that appropriate changes in management may be made.

Adjusting to a chronic, lifelong disease comes next. How do you adjust? Do you ever completely adjust? How does stress affect the body, blood-glucose levels, and control of diabetes? Are you taking any vitamins, minerals, or herbs? The more information you give your health professionals, the more they can help you. But what do you tell them? What happens when you don't tell them the truth, the whole truth, and nothing but the truth? Then there are your family members and friends. They need to know how best to support you, and you need to tell them how they can accomplish this task. Too much "smothering" is not good. Too much "this is your own problem" is also not good. And, in closing, is there hope? If so, what does this "hope" include? This book won't give you any false expectations but will tell you what to watch for in the visual media and in books, magazines, and pamphlets.

Some of the material presented will be controversial. It is the intent of the authors to stimulate thinking. It is also the intent of the authors to have each person and family member look at diabetes in the most logical way possible. Principles will be stressed rather than actual procedures. By this we mean the ideas that seem to hold true no matter what the differences of opinion as far as approaches to management are concerned.

The appendices provide quick reference. Needless to say, all things could not be included, but many listings of information are provided. We trust that what is included will be the most helpful to you.

As you, the person with diabetes, or you, the family member who has a person in your family with diabetes, progress in your knowledge and care, keep in mind the statement made in the computer world: "Garbage in; garbage out." What you share with the health professionals will assist you or your family member in getting the quality care that you need. If the quality of care is lacking in an education format, a method of communication format, a way to monitor your diabetes format, or a management program format, consider the need for a specialist. You may already have been referred to such a person. You may have a mild type of diabetes that is terrifically managed by your family physician. Or you may profit from contact with an allied health specialist such as a Certified Diabetes Educator (CDE) or a person Board Certified in Advanced Diabetes Management (BC-ADM). Continually be aware of your body needs and the responses your body has to your diabetes treatment.

The Diabetes Sourcebook is only an aid to assist you in meeting the goals of quality diabetes control. As you report the results of your blood-glucose level monitoring and, when appropriate, your urine ketone test results, be sure to provide enough information to your health professionals so that they can make appropriate decisions. Perhaps this book will help you to ask useful questions during your clinic visits or as you attend class. Perhaps this book will help you to keep better records so that you can get better information in return. Whatever this book may assist you in doing, above all may it direct you toward improved health and a happier life.

1

What Kind of Diabetes Do You Have?

Having diabetes is like learning
to think and act for the pancreas.

DOROTHEA SIMS

Diabetes is not a single disease with a single cause. Rather, it is a collection of diseases, some more difficult to control than others. All forms of diabetes involve a hormone (body regulator) from the pancreas called *insulin*. If you have diabetes, either you lack insulin (i.e., Type 1 diabetes) or you are not able to use your insulin properly (i.e., insulin resistance or Type 2 diabetes). The result is that instead of being stored for energy through the action of insulin, the foods you eat (primarily the starches and carbohydrates) raise your blood sugar to higher-than-normal levels. Without treatment, your blood sugar remains high and has the potential to adversely affect every organ and system in your body. With treatment, the insulin problem can be solved, and your blood sugar can be brought down or normalized so that the body is not damaged. A person with diabetes can thus remain healthy and look forward to a normal life span.

A Bit of History

Information written on ancient Egyptian papyrus described diabetes as a disease that caused a person to melt into the loins and the resulting urine to attract ants (because of the sugar content). The name itself indicates the loss of valuable body fluids: *diabetes* is from a Greek word meaning "to siphon." *Mellitus*, a Latin word, relates to a word meaning "honey" or "sweet tasting." Yes, due to the high sugar content and the lack of earlier testing methodologies, actually tasting the urine did give an indication that the person had sugar diabetes! In fact, Mother Nature was fooling the disease's early observers, who saw the crystalline content of the urine after its liquid contents had evaporated. In the fourteenth century, this was actually thought to be a salt (people were not into taste-testing at that time, we suppose).

Diabetes mellitus was treated, over time, by various means aimed at lowering the sugar content in the urine or decreasing the loss of fluid. Some patients fasted and feasted on alternating days, weeks, or months. Others were taught to eat rancid meat or vegetables cooked three times in their own water. Others survived on eggs or cereal. The association of food and fluid was passed down through time. Eventually, the discovery was made that the hormone insulin, secreted by cells called beta cells in the islets of Langerhans, needed to be replaced in the body in order for normal blood-glucose levels to be achieved.

Many people contributed to the knowledge about monitoring blood-glucose levels. Insulin could not be analyzed or its significant content noted until the 1960s. We learned that other hormones, such as glucagon, might help cause the disease. We also learned that diabetes is not the result of a single event in the body but of several events that lead to a series of immune responses, with the end result being that the majority of insulin-making beta cells no longer work.

With the discovery of insulin, many people believed that diabetes had been cured. The medical community soon discovered, however, that if the person lived longer, and especially when the blood-glucose levels were not significantly controlled or normalized the majority of the time, complications occurred (for example, blindness, heart disease, or the need for amputation). Many of these complications can now be prevented through present knowledge of this process or by getting to the doctor in time. Eyes (retinopathy) are being stabilized and vision returned (a risk reduction of 76 percent).

In one case, a young man had 350/20 vision in the right eye, 400/20 in the left eye, a detached retina in the left eye, cataract development in both eyes, and cloudy fluid in the eyes due to past hemorrhages. With the lasering of the total retina surface, a procedure that reattached the retina to the back surface of the eye, replacement of the eye fluid, and lens removal and implant of a new lens, vision improved to 40/20 in the right eye and 30/20 in the left eye.

Amputation, a procedure most associated with diabetes in its earlier days, can be prevented in an increasing number of cases (risk reduction of nerve disease, or neuropathy: 60 percent). Other problems associated with other parts of the body are reversed earlier or treated with transplantation (e.g., risk reduction of kidney disease, or nephropathy: 53 percent), something unheard of twenty-five or more years ago.

Education of the diabetes patient is one of the major keys to attaining such high degrees of control. Since health professionals cannot be with the person and his or her family on a day-in, day-out basis, self-management education is a must. Demand it.

Types of Diabetes

Diabetes has been divided into three groups: Type 1, or insulin-dependent diabetes mellitus, for which insulin must be injected daily; Type 2, or insulin-resistant diabetes mellitus, for which insulin injections are usually not necessary; and secondary diabetes (due to pancreatic surgery or overactive glands, such as the pituitary or the adrenals). We are concerned here only with Type 1 and Type 2 diabetes.

Type 1 diabetes is believed to be caused by a combination of genetics and environmental stressors. The individual who develops Type 1 diabetes has an inability to make insulin. When insulin is absent, the cells are in a state of starvation, while an excess of sugar in the form of glucose is available in the blood. This state of high blood-glucose levels is called hyperglycemia or, in this case, diabetes mellitus. (Hyperglycemia may be caused by a number of stressors, but when it is due to problems with insulin it is called diabetes mellitus.) Despite eating vast amounts of food the person remains in a condition of starvation until adequate insulin is available and can get the food into the cells. Body fat is burned as an alternate fuel to sugar; a by-product, ketone bodies, is created as a source of energy. But ketones cause the accumulation of acids and upset the body's buffer system. The body develops a serious problem known as ketoacidosis, a chemical imbalance of the body accompanied by high blood sugar and excess acid. This creates the classic symptoms of out-of-control diabetes: frequent urination (polyuria), excessive thirst (polydipsia), and excessive hunger (polyphagia). If neglected, ketoacidosis can eventually lead to death.

Type 2 diabetes, also called non-insulin-dependent diabetes, has been known by many other names, such as maturity onset diabetes, insulin-resistant diabetes, nonketosis prone, ketosis resistant, and even MODY, or Maturity Onset Diabetes in the Young. Eighty to 85 percent of the diabetes population is diagnosed as having Type 2 diabetes. Of these diabetics, 88 percent or so are overweight. Many of the so-called borderline diabetics are Type 2s who have been mislabeled. Overweight children may have Type 2 diabetes.

Insulin is still the key factor in this disease, but often there is an excess rather than a lack. The increase in insulin is believed to be the result of resistance. The excess insulin causes or results from the inability to use available receptor sites (that is, links to get the insulin into the cell). In the absence of or inability of receptor sites to function well (i.e., work with the available insulin), the result is diabetes (hyperglycemia). While the elevation in blood-glucose levels may lead to polyuria, polydipsia, and polyphagia, as in Type 1 diabetes, a key difference exists.

Insulin is the key factor in all forms of diabetes. In the case of Type 1 diabetes the problem is the lack of insulin. With Type 2 diabetes there may, at least early in the course of the disease, be an excess of the hormone. The cause of this excess is not entirely understood, but is due at least in part to inherited characteristics interacting with some lifestyle problems. The life problems are aging, obesity, and inactivity.

Though the inheritance for Type 2 diabetes is probably widespread through all peoples of the world, the disease is more frequently seen as the income of the country increases. This is due to the insulin resistance that may be triggered from the excess food intake and decreased energy expenditure that results in obesity. When there is obesity in persons who have the inheritance for diabetes (Type 2), for some reason the insulin does not work right for the muscle and fat cells (insulin resistance), and the pancreas must then produce more insulin to get the same result. This excess insulin production ultimately leads to exhaustion of the insulin-producing cells, which leads to decreased production. Now we have two defects: insulin resistance with increased insulin need, and insulin deficiency due to lack of production. Either outcome will result in increased blood sugar and the diagnosis of diabetes mellitus. Polyuria, polydipsia, and polyphagia symptoms are very prominent in

Type 1 diabetes but may or may not be present in Type 2 diabetes until very late in the course of the disease when there is a marked lack of insulin.

In Type 1 diabetes there is a lack of insulin, and polyphagia is usually accompanied by weight loss, but with Type 2 diabetes there more likely will be weight gain. The major function of insulin is storage of excess food, so the weight gain is easily understandable. Overeating and insulin resistance lead to excess insulin production that results in the storage of excess food, causing more fat, which causes more insulin resistance and more insulin secretion, which stores more food, and so on. Decreasing food intake and increasing energy expenditure (exercising) to reduce obesity and take the strain off the pancreas to produce extra insulin are vital to treating this disease.

The cause of the insulin resistance is not known. We know there is an inherited defect, but its actual identity is not known. Indeed there may be many inherited defects that can cause insulin resistance in the presence of obesity. These defects may include a defect in the number or shape of the chemicals on the cell membrane that accepts the insulin (called a receptor) or a variety of defects that can occur inside the cell so that the insulin cannot work properly. Many possible defects have been identified, so there can be many kinds of Type 2 diabetes. All the defects appear to have some relation to obesity as the precipitating phenomenon leading to insulin resistance, excess insulin production, beta cell exhaustion, and decreased insulin production (insulin deficiency). The result is high blood sugar that itself can be toxic to the insulin-producing cells (glucose toxicity) and further damage them, leading to a greater decrease in insulin production, more insulin deficiency, and more increase in the blood sugar—resulting in a vicious cycle. Treatment should occur as early as possible to preserve the beta cell function and insulin production.

Type 1 diabetes is most often diagnosed in children, with a peak incidence during the preadolescent growth spurt. The disease can occur at any age and must never be misdiagnosed just because the person is older. Type 2 diabetes is more common in people over the age of thirty-five, but it can also occur at any age. We are in fact seeing an increase in this form of the disease in children, associated with an increase in obesity of our children. People with newly diagnosed Type 1 diabetes have a tendency to be thin and to have lost weight. People with Type

2 diabetes are usually obese and will have gradually gained weight. Both types may require insulin for treatment. Type 1 patients are insulin dependent, i.e., they will die without the hormone replacement, while Type 2s may require insulin to control the blood sugar but will not die soon without it, although they can develop long-term complications that ultimately could be fatal. Sometimes these two forms of diabetes are difficult to tell apart. Some tests can be done to differentiate them, but these tests can be expensive, and family history and symptoms are more often used and are usually effective in differentiating the two types.

In 1997, new criteria for diagnosis and classification terminology were developed. These criteria are shown in Tables 1.1 and 1.2. All diabetes is diagnosed by one of three criteria: (1) a fasting plasma glucose level (FPG) of 126 mg/dl or 7 mmol (the measure used in most countries other than the USA—the conversion factor is 18) on two occasions; (2) a value of 200 mg/dl or 11.1 mmol at two hours after an oral glucose load (rarely used anymore); or (3) a random value greater than 200 mg/dl or 11 mmol if accompanied by symptoms usually associated with diabetes. These are the criteria that should be used today for diagnosis of all patients. If the FPG is greater than normal (110 mg/dl–6 mmol) but less than 126 mg/dl–7 mmol, or the two-hour value on the oral glucose tolerance test is greater than 140 mg/dl–7.08 mmol, but less than 199 mg/dl–11 mmol, the diagnosis is prediabetes. We no longer use the term *borderline diabetic*, which used to be used for these intermediate states, since that term has no meaningful criteria and is subject to any physician's interpretation. The above terms have precise definitions and are the same from doctor to doctor.

Type 1 diabetes has two subcategories: (1) autoimmune and (2) idiopathic. By this we mean that class 1 are of known cause in that there is absolute insulin deficiency caused by a defect in the immune system that destroys the beta cells of the pancreas. Idiopathic means that some other cause, such as removal of the pancreas, has occurred. Other specific types relate to the destruction of the pancreas by infection, inflammation, or chemicals, or some unknown cause that has destroyed the beta cells or the entire pancreas, so again there is complete insulin deficiency but not from destruction by the immune system. Type 2 diabetes can be subclassed as well, but the subclasses are still being developed. Most are adult and most are obese. An additional classification is gestational diabetes, which will be discussed later. See Table 1.2 for the criteria for

Table 1.1 Etiologic Classification of Diabetes Mellitus

I. Type 1 Diabetes (Beta cell destruction, usually leading to absolute insulin deficiency)
   A. Immune mediated
   B. Idiopathic

II. Type 2 Diabetes (May range from predominantly insulin resistant with relative insulin deficiency to a predominantly secretory defect with insulin resistance)

III. Other Specific Types
   A. Genetic defects of beta cell function:
      1. Chromosome 12, HNF-1 alpha (formerly MODY3)
      2. Chromosome 7, glucokinase (formerly MODY2)
      3. Chromosome 20, HNF-4 alpha (formerly MODY1)
   B. Genetic defects insulin action:
      1. Type A insulin resistance
      2. Leprechaunism
      3. Rabson-Mendenhall syndrome
      4. Lipoatophic diabetes
   C. Diseases of the exocrine pancreas:
      1. Pancreatitis
      2. Trauma/pancreatectomy
      3. Neoplasia
      4. Cystic fibrosis
      5. Hemochromatosis
      6. Fibrocalculous pancreatopathy
   D. Endocrinopathies:
      1. Acromegaly
      2. Cushing's syndrome
      3. Glucagonoma
      4. Pheochromocytoma
      5. Hyperthyroidism
      6. Somatostatinoma
      7. Aldosteronoma
   E. Drug or chemical induced:
      1. Vacor
      2. Pentamidine
      3. Nicotinic acid
      4. Glucocorticoids
      5. Thyroid hormone
      6. Diazoxide
      7. Beta adrenergic agonists
      8. Thiazides
      9. Dilantin
      10. Alpha interferon
   F. Infections:
      1. Congenital rubella
      2. Cytomegalovirus
   G. Uncommon forms of immune-medicated diabetes:
      1. "Stiff-man" syndrome
      2. Anti-insulin receptor antibodies
   H. Other genetic syndromes sometimes associated with diabetes

IV. Gestational Diabetes

Table 1.2 Classification of Diabetes

Stage	Fasting Plasma Glucose	Casual Plasma Glucose (random)	Two-hour Plasma Glucose
Diabetes	> or = 126 mg/dl (7.0 mmol)	> or = 200 mg/dl (11.1 mmol + symptoms)	> or = 200 mg/dl
Impaired Glucose Homeostasis	126 mg/dl	> 200 mg/dl (1 hour)	> or = 40–199 mg/dl
Normal	< 110 mg/dl	< 180 mg/dl (1 hour)	< 140 mg/dl

Report of the Expert Committee on the Diagnosis and Classification of Diabetes Mellitus. *Diabetes Care* 20(7) 1997, 1183–97.

impaired fasting glucose (IFG) or impaired glucose tolerance (IGT), which was renamed impaired glucose homeostasis, and is now named prediabetes.

Problems Associated with Diabetes

With Type 1 (insulin-dependent) diabetes, after the acute episode (diabetic ketoacidosis) or early symptoms leading to the diagnosis (frequent passing of urine, excess eating with weight loss, extreme thirst), there may be a partial remission period (the honeymoon) during which the body appears to be able to make some insulin again. This period usually lasts from three to six months, but it may last longer depending on the suppression of the insulin-making ability of the beta cells through an external insulin-injection program. Illness, poor blood sugar control, or extreme emotional stress appear to aid in further destruction of the beta cells, as does growth, and may shorten the remission period.

Eventually, the person becomes totally insulin dependent, especially if more than 90 percent of the beta cells become inactive. Except during the honeymoon or period of partial remission, people with Type 1 diabetes cannot make insulin. There will be no measurable insulin levels except of that which is injected and no measurable levels of any of the by-products of internal insulin secretion, such as a protein called

C-Peptide, which can differentiate internal and external insulin when it is present. The C-Peptide is present in persons with Type 2 diabetes, often in large amounts consistent with the elevated insulin levels, and can be used to differentiate Type 1 diabetes from Type 2. As time goes on and insulin secretion is decreased in Type 2 diabetes, C-Peptide will decrease as well and make this tool useless to differentiate the different kinds of diabetes. The C-Peptide test is expensive and not of much value except in a research setting.

2

Who Gets This Disease?

Diabetes mellitus is rapidly becoming an epidemic. The National Diabetes Data Group reported that from 1996 to 2000, the diagnosis of this disease increased 47 percent. Over eighteen million people in this country (8.9 percent of the population) have diabetes. Of this number, it is estimated that one-third more million people have this disease but have not been diagnosed. Worldwide, more than 183 million people currently have diabetes. The World Health Organization has projected that this figure will rise to 300 million by 2025. In *Diabetes 2001 Vital Statistics*, it was estimated that 27,000 new cases of diabetes per day were being diagnosed (90 percent of these people had Type 2 diabetes). The total number increased to an estimated 798,000 by the year 2000.

Diabetes is considered the fourth highest cause of death in most developed countries and the sixth-leading cause of death by disease in the United States. The ravages of this disease are blindness, or retinopathy (each year 12,000 to 24,000 diabetes people lose their sight); kidney disease, or nephropathy (more than 27,900 individuals develop end-stage kidney disease or kidney failure); nerve disease, or neuropathy, and amputations (more than 56,000 amputations are performed each year); and heart disease, or cardiovascular disease, and stroke (more than 77,000 deaths due to heart disease occur each year). Over 400,000 people, directly or indirectly, die from causes related to diabetes. The good news is that if blood-glucose levels are normal or near normal most of the time (as noted by a hemoglobin A1c—the amount of glucose that attaches to the protein of the red blood cell over a two-to-three-month period—of less than 7 percent), there is approximately a 76 percent reduced risk of developing retinopathy, a 53 percent reduced risk of developing nephropathy, a 60 percent reduced risk of developing neuropathy, and a potential 35 percent reduced risk of developing cardiovascular disease.

Health care costs the average person, who is not diabetic, over $2,000 per year. If the person has diabetes, this cost is $13,000 per year (both direct and indirect costs). Supplies alone cost $2,000 plus per year; if the person is using an insulin infusion pump, the cost jumps to $2,500 and higher.

The overall cost of the disease is rising rapidly. The total cost of diabetes in 1997 was estimated by the American Diabetes Association to be $98 billion. Now, some estimates have ranged as high as $132 billion. This number represents 10 percent of the total health care expenditure, and the higher number represents 15 percent of the health care dollar. The latter figure indicates that while diabetes afflicts only one out of every seventeen people, it takes one out of every seven health care dollars. Yet diabetes receives less than 1 percent of the national research budget or less than one out of every 100 research dollars. This is a serious problem that must be challenged if we are to find a cure and end this costly disease. We need to get the message to Congress that they need to reexamine priorities and allocate the proper proportion of the research budget to diabetes. "As bad as these bare numbers are, we must also remember that those who suffer losses due to diabetes are not just statistics on a chart. They are people whose talents and wisdom are needed and whose problems deserve our unified efforts. Together we can join to make life more just and more joyful for generations to come." This quote comes from Dr. David Satcher, former director of the Centers for Disease Control and former surgeon general of the United States.

While the numbers are bad, there is hope. Progress is being made, and life for people with diabetes gets better each day. It is the intent of this book to help you achieve that fuller and more joyful life even though you may have diabetes. It can be done. We as health professionals will try to help. Education of people with diabetes is one way to improve control of diabetes and quality of life and even save money. Many studies have reported great cost savings—as much as $3 million per year in one program (Miller, 1982)—through patient teaching and proper medical care.

Early Forms of Diabetes

Once called chemical diabetes, or prediabetes, early forms of carbohydrate intolerance include impaired glucose tolerance (IGT) and impaired fasting glucose (IFG), which are now called impaired glucose homeostasis (IGH). Impaired glucose homeostasis is the diagnosis for a person with a fasting glucose level greater than 100 but less than 126 mg/dl (7 mmol). It is also the diagnosis for a person who has a normal fasting blood sugar (glucose) and who, after drinking a certain amount of liquid that contains glucose (75 g), has a value at two hours of between 140 to 199 mg/dl (7.7 to 11 mmol). (The measurement *mmol* is metric; to convert mg/dl to mmol for blood sugar, divide by 18. For example: 200 mg/dl $\div$ 18 = 11.1 mmol.

Insulin values may be low, normal, or high, or in many cases have a delay in release. The delayed release may then lead to an excess release of insulin. The result of the delayed insulin release is a late drop in blood sugar, called reactive hypoglycemia.

Gestational Diabetes

Gestational diabetes develops during pregnancy and may revert back to impaired glucose homeostasis or previous abnormality of glucose tolerance after the pregnancy is over. It is possible that the female will progress to Type 1 diabetes or, more commonly, Type 2. Further testing is needed if the fasting blood-sugar level is above 105 mg/dl (5.8 mmol), or if a two-hour postmeal (postprandial) blood-sugar level is greater than 150 mg/dl (8 mmol).

It is recommended that high-risk pregnant females be screened, and they may need to be screened earlier than the twenty-fourth week of gestation. Screening before this date should be done on any pregnant female who may be suspect. Statistics show that prepregnancy control of blood-sugar (glucose) levels among pregnant diabetic women leads to mother and infant outcomes that are nearly the same as those for nondiabetic pregnant women. If control is achieved only by the second trimester, there is a 14 percent chance that the infant will die or develop complications, such as heart, head, or spinal malformations. The mother will have more problems with toxemia and eclampsia, such as that associated with inflammation of the pancreas (pancreatitis). The second trimester is the time during which the stresses of pregnancy begin to develop, and these effects elevate the blood-sugar levels. Treatment should begin promptly and continue from early in the pregnancy to the end.

Secondary Types of Diabetes

Secondary types of diabetes are due to a number of causes or states, such as injury to or surgical removal of the pancreas. Additional causes are associated with inflammation of the pancreas (pancreatitis) or elevated plasma iron associated with an enlarged liver, pigmentation of the skin, and (frequently) cardiac failure. Hormonal diseases such as Cushing's disease (puffy red face) or acromegaly (large face, long arms and hands) may also cause diabetes. Certain syndromes (for example, Prader-Willi, Down's, Progeria, and Turner's) may result in a hyperglycemic state; if this state is prolonged, the result can be permanent diabetes. Drugs such as steroids, Dilantin, and others may elevate the blood sugar through a variety of mechanisms. Certain other drugs, such as alloxan, streptozocin, and thiazide diuretics, are toxic to the beta cells of the pancreas and can cause diabetes.

Type 1 and Type 2 Diabetes

Diabetes resulting in an insulin-dependent state is classified as Type 1 diabetes. While Type 1 diabetes affects only 5 to 10 percent of the diabetic population, its effects on the body can be worse than from other forms of diabetes. In the past, Type 1 has been known as juvenile or juvenile-onset diabetes (because it is usually diagnosed in those under thirty), brittle diabetes, unstable diabetes, insulin-dependent diabetes, and ketosis-prone diabetes. People in this classification more frequently exhibit the classic symptoms, usually with ketones present in blood and urine. A blood-sugar level of 800 mg/dl (44 mmol) or higher, especially if ketones are not present, indicates a diagnosis of hyperglycemic hyperosmolar nonketotic syndrome, a state in which the body is extremely dry (dehydrated), the chemicals in the body are concentrated, and the blood sugar is high.

As stated before, diabetes is a syndrome or group of diseases (rather than one disease) leading to a prolonged hyperglycemic state. Type 1 is most associated with the killing of the beta cells, most likely by the body's own immune system. Either the immune system cannot kill an infecting agent, which then kills the beta cells, or the immune system itself goes "wild," attacking the body's own tissue and destroying the beta cells. The cells of the islets of Langerhans become inflamed, resulting from an infectious-disease process (for example, mumps) or, more commonly, from an autoimmune (allergic to self) response.

The autoimmune process results in the circulation of antibodies that may either cause or be caused by beta-cell death. If it is found that the antibodies cause beta-cell destruction (the body fighting what it now considers foreign to itself), the body's response to the Type 1 diabetes is much less severe (i.e., easier to control) with treatment. Until then, the outcome is a lack of available insulin. While the onset is said to be sudden, changes resulting in decreased insulin availability may have occurred over a longer period of time. In short, insulin-dependent diabetes mellitus is an inherited defect of the body's immune system, resulting in destruction of the insulin-producing beta cells of the pancreas.

Heredity is a major cause of diabetes. If both parents have Type 2 diabetes, there is a 100 percent chance that nearly all of their children will have diabetes, but in reality only 50 percent do. If both parents have Type 1 diabetes, fewer than 20 percent of their children will develop Type 1 diabetes. In identical twins, if one twin develops Type 2 diabetes, the chance is nearly 100 percent that the other twin will also develop it. With Type 1 diabetes, however, only 40 to 50 percent of the second twins will develop the disease, indicating that while inheritance is important, environmental factors (for example, too much food, too much stress, viral infection) are also involved in the development of diabetes.

Causes of Type 1 Diabetes

Type 1 diabetes is an inherited defect of the immune system triggered by an environmental stimulus or stimuli. The problem may be with the "on switch" of the immune system, with viral stimuli not activating the system. The virus is then allowed to penetrate the beta cells and cause their destruction. Alternatively, the problem may be with the "off switch." The system turns on appropriately and kills the virus but then does not turn itself off. The T-cells, defined as cells that "eat" germs, are then allowed to attack the beta cells. This is a very simplified explanation. In point of fact, the process is much more complex, involving many, many steps in the immune system. The beta cells themselves may contribute to the process by producing antigens or chemicals on the cell surface that stimulate the immune system, and there may be many other environmental stimuli besides viruses. Indeed, there is some evidence now that protein in certain types of cows' milk may cause the formation of antibodies that can attach to the beta cells or that are similar to antibodies on the beta cells. When the immune system mobilizes in response to a stimulus, these antibodies will attach to receptors on the surface of the beta cells, causing damage to occur to the beta cells of the pancreas. For whatever reason, the beta cells are then destroyed by the immune system in what is called an autoimmune phenomena, in which the body has come to identify itself as a foreign body and begins to eliminate certain parts.

Recently researchers have been attempting to locate the genes for diabetes. As part of the genome project, in which researchers around the world attempted to map the entire gene structure of all the human chromosomes, they isolated more than eighteen genes that appear to be involved in the production of Type 1 diabetes. Not all of these genes have equal potency. Two of them appear to be very potent, some others are less potent, and others are simply auxiliary or helper genes that seem to have some assisting effect in the process. There are also genes that are protective, so that if one inherited the genes for diabetes but also inherited the protective genes, one would not develop the disease. Thus, development of the disease is not 100 percent likely in those who have inherited the genetics for the disease. Some people may have the genes, but they may also either have protector genes or be fortunate enough to avoid the environmental stimuli.

The cause of Type 1 diabetes, then, is an inherited defect in the immune system that interacts in some way with environmental factors. These factors may be viruses or chemicals in the environment, or perhaps other environmental factors that we have not yet identified, that team up and eventually result in the complete destruction of the beta cells and the loss of insulin secretion.

Causes of Type 2 Diabetes

The causes of Type 2 diabetes, besides the genetic factor, are not as well understood. Two factors appear to be important in Type 2 diabetes. These are insulin resistance and insulin deficiency. There is a debate over which comes first, but the general consensus of the moment is that insulin resistance is the first factor. Type 2 diabetes is also a genetic disease, although the genes are carried, for the most part, on entirely different chromosomes than those for Type 1 diabetes. There are probably multiple genes involved in this disease. For whatever reason, this genetic factor, perhaps interacting with some environmental factors such as excess caloric intake, deficient caloric expenditure, and aging, may result in a resistance to insulin. That is, the peripheral cell, a muscle or fat or other cell, does not respond appropriately to the insulin present. The body then begins to produce more insulin in order to try to overcome the insulin resistance.

The next part of the sequence may involve two factors. One is that the increasing insulin secretion may ultimately exhaust the beta cells, thus resulting in insulin deficiency. Another factor has been identified recently—glucose toxicity. It turns out that sugar in high amounts can be toxic or poisonous to the cells of the body. In persons with insulin resistance who are running high blood sugars that have been undetected and untreated, or in the person who knows he or she has the disease but does not treat it appropriately, the continuing high levels of sugar have a toxic effect on the insulin-producing cells of the pancreas, thus damaging those cells and reducing insulin secretion. So we then end up with a combination of peripheral resistance to the action of insulin and, at the same time, insulin deficiency. Those two conditions can then precipitate a severe case of Type 2 diabetes that may in fact require insulin for treatment.

There are many steps in the action of insulin at the peripheral cell level, and each of those steps is stimulated by a different enzyme, and each enzyme is controlled by a different gene. Therefore, there are many potential places where the defects can occur, resulting in the same ultimate end: resistance of the peripheral cells to the action of insulin. This is probably the precipitating factor in Type 2 diabetes.

Facts and Figures

Both Type 1 and Type 2 diabetes are increasing in the population, but there is a more pronounced increase in Type 2. The rate of increase of the disease is about 9 percent per year, which means the number of people with diabetes will double every eleven years. In the United States this increase is occurring predominately in the nonwhite ethnic populations. The prevalence of diabetes in the Caucasian population is approximately 5 to 6 percent; in the African American population it is somewhere between 12 and 15 percent; in the Hispanic population it is around 20 percent; and in the Native American population it frequently exceeds 30 percent. Indeed, there are tribes in which the prevalence may be as high as 65 percent.

Likewise, diabetes is increasing around the world, particularly in developing countries. However, the disease is very rare in third world or undeveloped countries. But as these countries begin to develop and achieve industrial prominence and economic stability, the cases of diabetes occurring in these cultures mushrooms. This was seen in Japan after World War II and most recently in Korea and Taiwan, and it is now occurring in other Southeast Asian countries as the standard of living begins to rise. It is thought that this increase is probably related to increased caloric intake associated with decreased caloric expenditure. The genes for Type 2 diabetes are probably widespread throughout the world in equal amounts for all races and ethnic groups. The change in lifestyle from manual labor with a low caloric intake to industrial labor with a high caloric intake and reduced caloric expenditure, because of the use of machinery, can result in a virtual explosion of Type 2 diabetes.

Type 1 diabetes is prevalent in certain geographic areas that are close to the equator, and as one moves farther north to the arctic circle the prevalence of the disease increases. The highest incidence occurs in the Scandinavian countries; the lowest occurs in the Mediterranean area, except for the island of Sardinia, which has an incidence equal to that of Finland. The reasons for these differences are not well understood, but it is believed to be due to obtaining milk from Brahman cows rather than Northern European cows (Jerseys, Guernseys, Holsteins, etc.). It is believed that there may be, in these cows used throughout Europe and the western hemisphere, a protein that may somehow cause damage to the pancreas and that this protein is lacking in the milk of Brahman cows usually found in Africa and Asia. Time and research will tell if this is truly a causative factor in Type 1 diabetes in Europe and North America.

3

How Is Diabetes Treated?

The treatment of diabetes mellitus must be varied from person to person and from time to time. The goals of treatment are listed in Table 3.1.

A variety of things affect the treatment of this disease for each individual. There are, for example, personal changes, such as changing jobs, moving, and taking on new responsibilities. There is a change in response from morning to noon, and from noon to midnight. If a person is highly stressed, there is going to be a difference. If a person is relaxed, there is going to be a difference. The type of diabetes will also make a difference. (Note that a person who does not have diabetes will have very little change in blood sugar even after eating a whole box of candy, but the person with diabetes will have elevated blood-sugar levels.) The following sections describe some of these differences and tell you how you can share this information with your health professional.

Differences in Treatment for Children and Adults

A child cannot be treated as a miniature adult. A one-unit change in insulin in a forty-pound child will have much more of an effect than a one-unit change in a 140-pound adult. Children not only have rapidly changing size but also rapidly changing hormones. These changing hormones lead to various changes in emotional responses. In some children

Table 3.1 Ideal Versus Acceptable Blood Sugars

Blood-sugar Goals	Ideal	Acceptable	American Association of Clinical Endocrinologists
Fasting blood sugar	70–110 mg/dl (3.8/6.1 mmol)	60–120 mg/dl (3.3–6.6 mmol)	<110 (6.1 mmol)
1 hour after meal	90–150 mg/dl (5.0–8.3 mmol)	80–180 mg/dl (4.4–10.0 mmol)	———
2 hours after meal	80–140 mg/dl (4.4–7.7 mmol)	70–150 mg/dl (3.8–8.3 mmol)	<140 (7.7 mmol)
3 hours after meal	60–100 mg/dl (3.3–5.5 mmol)	60–130 mg/dl (3.3–7.2 mmol)	———
Hemoglobin A1c	6%	<7%	<6.5%

Average blood sugars for a pregnant woman with diabetes should be around 90 mg/dl (5 mmol).

with Type 1 diabetes, the disease is more severe; if beta-cell function is preserved, it may be milder. More food is needed for a child's active lifestyle, as well as for growth and development. More food means the need of more insulin.

As with any type of diabetes, the goal is to attain and maintain a high degree of control of blood-glucose levels and a quality of life that makes it all worthwhile. If a child does not get enough to eat and enough insulin to help get food into the cells for energy and growth, he or she will not grow at all or will not grow at the rate expected.

If blood sugars are normalized most of the time, the only time a child should ever be ill with diabetes is at diagnosis, when diabetic ketoacidosis (high blood-glucose levels, dehydration, and chemical [electrolyte] imbalance) is present. Learning when to give more insulin for higher blood sugars prevents diabetic ketoacidosis from ever occurring again.

Often, diabetic ketoacidosis (DKA) can be predicted (for example, if there is an infection). More fluids and more insulin, as needed, would keep a DKA problem from occurring. Checking for ketones in the urine would tell the parents whether the child's body is using fats as an energy source. If the blood-glucose levels are high (300 mg/dl [17 mmol] or greater), the body can become chemically out of balance and the child can become very sick.

Low blood-glucose levels (hypoglycemia or insulin reaction) are the other side of the coin. This condition is a little more difficult to handle. Some people are more afraid of the short-term effects of low blood sugar than the long-term effects of high blood sugar. Some occurrences of hypoglycemia can be predicted—for example, if a child is anticipating something special the next day and so is not sleeping well. If they can be predicted, then in most cases they can be prevented. If they are not predicted, rapid and early treatment is most helpful. If the symptoms or feelings are ignored or are not noticeable enough, a problem could occur.

Blood-glucose testing has been a great help in the early detection of low blood sugar. Small children may not have the words to say that they are "feeling funny." Or they might be so involved in play that they do not notice that their falling blood sugars are giving them signals that it's time to get something to eat. If they feel hunger, there is more of a chance they will respond by getting something to eat, but this is not always so.

A mild insulin reaction now and then is nothing compared to frequent times of very low blood-glucose levels. The brain can take only so much, such as the lack of a fuel source, before it will undergo cell damage. This is especially true if the reactions are of the severe type (jerking or unconsciousness). *Severe reactions must be prevented at all costs.* Occasional mild episodes of shaking and sweating, although somewhat uncomfortable to experience, are not as serious as severe reactions. If the child has not reached the age of full nerve development (six to eight years of age), there is a greater chance that severe hypoglycemia will result in brain damage.

Allowing anyone—child or adult—to have high blood sugar (hyperglycemia) all the time is also not recommended. The person will be dull, less alert, and often more irritable. Teachers and employers will usually report a change in learning or working ability when the blood sugar is either too high or too low. True, the child or adult is not having insulin reactions, but, in the long term, a slight insulin reaction now and then is much less damaging than chronic high blood-glucose levels. Interestingly, if the blood-glucose control is poor, there is often a greater chance of having severe insulin reactions.

The chance of having more severe insulin reactions with higher blood-glucose content has been debated. The Diabetes Control and Complications Trial, a ten-year study to determine what level of control very early on will best reduce the risk of having complications, stated that the more normal the glucose control, the greater the chance of having severe insulin reactions. In the third year of the study, the intensive control group experienced a 30 to 40 percent increase in low blood-glucose levels compared to the standard control group. Most of the first group's hypoglycemia was without symptoms, with blood-glucose values in the forties. A year later, at the national meeting of the American Diabetes Association, it was announced that there had been a change in treatment methods and that hypoglycemia in their population had decreased. As a side comment, the speaker said he guessed they were learning how to manage diabetes better because there were fewer low blood-glucose reactions in the intensive control group. Our own experience has been that the number of severe hypoglycemic episodes is fewer, or certainly no greater, among children or adults in "tighter" control than among those with wildly swinging or chronically high blood sugars.

As diabetic ketoacidosis is usually associated with infection or prolonged emotional stress, so hypoglycemia is associated with a mistake in the amount of insulin given, a lot of play or exercise without extra food, or manipulation of food (for example, a child's refusal to eat food in order to get his or her way). This is why education and the type of treatment program chosen are so helpful.

Part of a parent's education includes the following: The total daily dose of insulin divided into multiple doses per day spreads out the impact of the peak, or top, action of the insulin. If you give all the insulin in one dose, unless it is Glargine (with a longer duration of action), it won't cover the entire twenty-four-hour time period; in addition, the strongest action time of the insulin might cause hypoglycemia then but cause hyperglycemia before the next dose is given. Spreading out the doses allows no great impact at any one time. Multiple doses don't mean that the diabetes is getting worse. It's just a method of allowing more flexibility in a lifestyle.

Psychological adjustment to the disease can develop when more flexibility is present. Children who have parents who support them often just take their diabetes in stride. Also, the younger child frequently adjusts more easily than does the teenager or the adult. Parents, on the other hand, may become too protective or may, either subconsciously or openly, reject the child. If the parents are not educated and supported by health care professionals, the child may become upset to the point that the diabetes becomes very hard to manage. Discipline becomes an extremely important part in the treatment program for the child. The more lovingly the child is disciplined, the greater the chance that he or she will have a long and healthy life.

When a group of children with diabetes was compared to a group of children without it, it was found that there was no greater number of conflicts or psychological diagnoses in one group than in the other. It was also noted that the diabetes management was poorer in families that did not work as a team.

Acute Care

The initial management of Type 1 diabetes is about the same for adults and children. Most physicians will give small amounts of insulin continuously or hourly in relation to the person's size and in relation to the state of ketoacidosis and dehydration. In fact, some intravenous fluids are usually given before insulin. Just think about this: If you have a glass half filled with water and you put ten teaspoons of sugar in it, would you have a faster response in lowering the amount of sugar in each teaspoon of liquid if you put in something to use up the sugar or if you filled the glass to the top with water? It's the same with the human body. Fluid is added, then insulin is started. When the laboratory work comes back, other chemicals such as potassium are added if necessary. Also, in some cases the doctor will not add the potassium until the person passes urine (otherwise, the potassium would become too concentrated in the body and cause problems).

The rate at which the blood-glucose levels fall is usually controlled so that it does not exceed much more than 100 mg/dl (5.5 mmol) per hour. This helps the body in its rebalancing process. It also helps prevent headaches, since the brain would otherwise get too much of a jolt by having the sudden greater amount of fluid and lesser amount of sugar. Saline, or salt water, may be given first, as it aids the tissues in accepting the fluid that is needed. Later on, glucose is added to the saline, or the total intravenous fluid is changed to a glucose solution. This may seem strange when the problem was initially caused by too much glucose in the system. However, the glucose in the water does a number of things. For one, it prevents the person from becoming hypoglycemic. For another, it prevents the person from making ketones from free fatty acids when the body recognizes that it needs something for energy.

To monitor the other chemicals in the body to be sure they are not out of balance, it is necessary to do blood tests every few hours. Usually, the blood is drawn through a plastic needle placed in a vein; to prevent clotting, very small amounts of heparin are put into the needle once the blood has been removed (this is called a "heparin lock"). Each time a specimen is needed, the heparin fluid is withdrawn, and the amount of blood needed is removed. Heparin is then put back into the needle space until the next specimen is needed. This procedure prevents the need to stick a person many times to obtain blood specimens. The plastic needle may be kept in place until the intravenous infusion (IV) is discontinued or after the first day or two (six to forty-eight hours).

Another way of testing how well a person is doing is by looking at the cardiac monitor. Not only can nurses and doctors tell whether chemicals such as potassium are at low or high levels, they can also tell whether calcium, magnesium, or other chemicals called electrolytes are out of balance. Actually, when there is adequate fluid replacement in the face of the appropriate amount of insulin, the other chemicals seem to balance out.

Management of Type 1 Diabetes

Depending on the management program you are on, once the acute state of the diabetes is controlled you may be discharged from the hospital and asked to return to the doctor on a daily, weekly, or monthly basis, plus receive some education on basic survival skills (how to administer the insulin, how to plan a meal, how to treat a reaction, how to monitor blood-glucose levels and urine ketones, and when and what to tell the doctor). You may be asked to return a few weeks or months later for more intensive education.

If the hospitalization time is short, the physician will start the total amount of daily insulin delivery at a lower level and increase the dosage until the suitable level of diabetes control is achieved. With a longer hospitalization, the physician will administer what is termed a "physiological amount of insulin," based on the patient's body size and food intake. The insulin is then lowered on a daily basis until the baseline, or normal, blood-glucose levels are stabilized.

Each method has its pros and cons. The former gives less early support, allowing the person to develop habits that might not be appropriate. But it does get the person back to work or school sooner and into a scheduled lifestyle from which individual needs can be assessed. The latter approach gives more initial psychological and physiological support. With this approach, most programs try to have the person's daily lifestyle mimicked by the activity and education program planned. This approach also appears to have a longer "honeymoon" period, during which the control of blood sugar may be easily obtained through the use of small amounts of insulin. This is due to the beta cells having recovered some ability to produce insulin internally. Research has shown that supporting internal beta cell function by giving some external insulin makes the diabetes easier to control for a longer period of time (from six months to three or four years).

Whatever the program, it needs to be individualized, with the person's lifestyle taken into account: When is exercise scheduled? When are the coffee breaks? What time is bedtime? When are meals usually eaten? The food should be patterned to meet the everyday needs. The insulin is then patterned to get the products of the food (such as glucose or proteins and, indirectly, fats) to go to the places they are supposed to go. As needs and age requirements change, the program must also change. If a person becomes more sedentary, the food intake needs to be decreased and the insulin (or oral agent, for adults) decreased. If too much insulin is given, the person could either have trouble with insulin reactions or may eat to compensate for the symptoms of hunger that occur with low blood sugar, and thus become overweight. As a child grows and requires more food (not just more carbohydrates, but more total calories), he or she will require more insulin. As the child becomes an adult, stops growing, and requires less food, less insulin will be required.

In the nondiabetic person, the body produces a small amount of insulin continuously. This is called *basal insulin*. The body then produces a burst of insulin after each intake of food (i.e. bolus). It is this pattern that must be duplicated for the diabetic, whatever treatment regimen is chosen. For people with Type 1, diabetes mellitus, this pattern can be duplicated in many ways, with many food patterns and insulin patterns (for example, five, four, three, or two doses of insulin per day). The minimum requirement for duplicating the normal pattern is three meals, with one to three between-meal and bedtime snacks, and an insulin pattern of two doses per day (before breakfast or supper) of a mixture of a short-acting (regular) or rapid-acting (lispro and aspart) insulin and an intermediate-acting insulin (NPH or lente) or long-acting insulin.

Intermediate-acting insulins last about twice as long as regular insulin, about twelve to fourteen hours, and half as long as long-acting insulin, such as ultralente or glargine. The two doses of intermediate-acting and the one or two doses of long-acting insulin provide the needed twenty-four-hour basal insulin and do a moderate job of supplying the bolus insulin for lunch (insulin to cover the immediate food intake). The added two doses of short-acting insulin with breakfast and supper provide the boluses or bursts for these meals. The two doses are given as mixed insulin before breakfast and before supper. In this method of management, usually twice as much insulin is given in the A.M. as in the P.M., because two meals are eaten in the A.M. and one meal in the P.M.

In many cases, indeed in most cases of Type 1 diabetes after the honeymoon or remission period, two shots per day are not enough. The most common problem is a high-fasting blood sugar in the morning upon arising. This is caused by the insulin taken at supper not lasting through the night. If we try to correct this by increasing the supper insulin dose we frequently cause nighttime low blood sugars that can have very bad consequences. A better solution to the problem is to split up the supper insulin and give only a short-acting or rapid-acting insulin before supper and give the intermediate-acting insulin (NPH or lente) at bedtime. In this regimen, you must test your blood sugar and make the appropriate corrections to the insulin doses.

Remember to:

1. Use the blood-sugar measurement after breakfast or prelunch to adjust the morning short- or rapid-acting insulin.
   The rapid-acting insulins are lispro (Humalog) and aspart (Novolog).
2. Use the blood-sugar measurement in the afternoon or presupper to adjust the morning NPH or lente insulin.

3. Use the after-supper blood-sugar measurement to adjust the supper insulin.
4. Use the fasting blood-sugar measurement in the morning to adjust the evening NPH or lente.

Lispro and aspart can be substituted for the short-acting insulin in a two-, three-, four-, or five-dose per day regimen. These insulins are taken with the meal instead of thirty minutes before, which adds convenience as well as better control, with fewer problems of low blood sugars. The dose of this insulin can be modified at the meal based on how much food is on the plate and can even be given after the meal, especially for small children with erratic eating patterns. These insulins are more physiologic since they are absorbed to better cover the blood sugar elevations as a result of the foods eaten. They peak in an hour or so and are gone in about two to three hours. These insulins, therefore, do not carry over to the next meal like regular insulin, which can cause premeal low blood sugars.

Flexibility, better control, and less low blood sugars makes these insulins very helpful for most people who need insulin. Remember, though, that these rapid-acting insulins are gone before the next meal, so the blood-sugar measurement must be taken two hours after the meal instead of before the next meal. A given blood-sugar measurement is then used to adjust the preceding insulin dose. Thus patterns of blood sugar are used to adjust the next day's dose instead of the next dose increased up or down or omitted as is done in sliding scale or other programs based on the immediate blood-glucose value.

Management of Type 2 Diabetes

For some adults with mild elevations of blood sugar, redistribution of calories throughout the day (just as insulin dosages are distributed throughout the day) keeps the body from being challenged at any one time of day and may aid in smoothing out the blood-sugar levels. If weight loss or choices of food do not aid the person in maintaining an average blood sugar below 150 mg/dl (8 mmol), then the person will need some oral agent to assist the body in functioning more appropriately. If an illness occurs during which a person cannot keep food down or the beta cells decrease their functioning, the person might temporarily need to go on insulin. Often, the oral agents will no longer work after five to ten years (this is called secondary failure of oral agents), and the person will need to start using insulin. Especially if it is determined that the person is insulin resistant and thus actually requires high doses of insulin, some health professionals find that they need to combine dosages of insulin with an oral agent given once or twice a day. (See Chapter 6 for more information.)

Exercise is a very important part of the adult's and child's management program. Ideally, children get needed exercise through planned programs in school. Adults must exercise on their own. Exercise offers many benefits, one of which is a greater sensitivity to insulin by the receptor sites of the cells.

As the adult ages, the management program changes again. If a complication of diabetes develops, many changes occur. If the problem involves the eyes, treatment will be needed to stabilize them. Adjusting to this treatment will likely cause changes in the person's activity pattern; emotions will thus be involved. If the problem involves the kidneys, blood pressure will need to be controlled. The use of medication to treat blood pressure may alter blood-glucose levels. If kidneys are affected by the aging process or by disease, the body will retain the insulin or oral-agent chemicals longer than is desired. There may thus be a need for lower doses of insulin or less of an oral agent, or a change from an oral agent to insulin.

As adults adjust to having diabetes and learn more about their own care, their diabetes control can truly be fine-tuned. The word *diabetes* does not need to be in neon lights all the time! Changes of lifestyle may seem like obstacles to anyone who has diabetes, but a better way to see them is as challenges that happen to accompany the diagnosis of diabetes.

Special Management Needs

Pregnancy

For the pregnant woman with Type 1, Type 2, or gestational diabetes, there are certain changes in the body's needs. Pregnancy has been called a "diabetogenic state." Pregnancy is stressful to the body, and anything that is stressful to the body results in the release of hormones that allow or cause the blood sugar to become elevated. The metabolic rate is higher, so the body burns food faster. Greater amounts of food are needed as the pregnancy progresses. As greater amounts of food are needed, more insulin is needed. Hormones produced by the placenta also increase insulin needs.

On delivery of the placenta, after the baby is born, the hormones that have resulted in high blood sugars are now no longer available to the body. Less insulin is then needed. Breast-feeding will further reduce the insulin need. If the female has diabetes only during pregnancy, it is possible that the blood-glucose levels will return to normal four to six weeks after delivery.

Although diabetes may be detected during a routine screening sometime during the twenty-fourth to twenty-eighth week of gestation, the pregnant woman may come to the doctor's office because she is feeling unusually tired—the result of high blood sugar. High blood sugar also results in blurry vision, sores that don't heal, and frequency of urination. Symptoms like those of the flu or appendicitis may be felt. Treatment to return the blood-glucose levels to normal makes these symptoms go away. During pregnancy, it is a must to keep blood sugars normal to prevent problems for both mother and baby. (See Chapter 10 for more information.)

Travel

Your health professional can help to prepare you for travel. Another resource is the International Travel Association. You may also call, E-mail, or check the website for the American Diabetes Association to get information about the names and addresses of physicians in almost any part of the world. You can also find out what equipment is available in various countries in case you run out of supplies (but try not to!). You should be able to say "I need a doctor" in the appropriate language. Traveling on planes and trains can be made much easier when you know what to eat, when to eat it, and whom to contact if special meals are desired. (Again, see Chapter 10 for more information.)

June Biermann and Barbara Toohey, the initial developers of the SugarFree Centers, are two people who have looked at life's obstacles as challenges. June has insulin-dependent diabetes, but this has never kept her from skiing the biggest mountain or exploring the farthest island. She has done this through self-management. Learning self-management means learning how your body responds to certain amounts of food, certain kinds of food, and certain amounts of diabetes medication. It also means knowing that if you have to take other medication for colds, flu, or other health problems, you plan for this with your health professional before you travel.

4

What About Education?

The more we learn about diabetes mellitus, the more complex it seems to become. Basic information is available that can assist the person who has diabetes to make this complex disease easier to understand. This information can be presented on three levels: a basic "survival" level, with just enough information to help the person (or family) in the completion of daily tasks; a home-management level, which includes the basics on almost all topics related to the disease; and a self-management level, which includes what a person needs to know for true self-management. Self-management involves decision making within a program that has been developed specifically for you by your physician or other qualified health care provider, such as a certified diabetes educator (CDE), a board certified advanced diabetes management (BC-ADM) nurse practitioner, a clinical nurse specialist, a pharmacist, or a dietitian.

Levels of Education

Basic "Survival" Level

The survival level of education includes what medication to take, how much of it to take, and when to take it. If you are giving yourself your own injections, you would be taught how to get the insulin into the syringe, how to administer the injection, and how to take care of your supplies and equipment. Guidance would be given in regard to nutritious food choices, the amounts to eat, and when they should be eaten. To keep track of yourself and to determine if what you are doing is correct, you would monitor your blood-glucose levels using a finger-stick test. If your blood-glucose levels were 250 mg/dl (13.8 mmol) or greater, you would be told to check your urine for ketones, especially if you were ill or taking insulin. Since below-normal blood-glucose levels might be a side effect of the administration of either oral hypoglycemic agents or insulin, you would be taught how to recognize low blood sugar and how to treat it. Most important, you would be taught when to contact your health professionals and what to tell them.

These are the basics, and they should be included as part of your management program before you leave the hospital or in conjunction with your initial visits to your doctor or other health care professional concerning your diabetes. You should always expect at least this minimum of education regarding your disease.

Home-Management Level

Home management goes beyond the above aspects of care. Not only do you learn more about the medication you are receiving, you also receive more detailed information on products and supplies. In addition, you learn about exercise and its integral role in your program. It is possible that you and your health professional will determine an exercise or increased activity program.

Hygiene is also a necessary part of home-management care. This hygiene involves care of the hair, the teeth, and the skin, with a specific emphasis on the feet for adults. Your feet get the most punishment of all your body parts and therefore need some special care. This care includes washing and inspecting your feet daily and wearing clean socks. Many problems can be avoided if a foot or skin infection is reported to your physician before it has a chance to become a real problem. Unless you have deep skin folds on the sides of your nails, cutting your toenails straight across (with the corners filed) prevents ingrown toenails and thus sites for infection. Stay away from hot-water bottles, heating pads, and sharp devices to protect those tender feet.

With home management, you will also learn what to do when you travel, go on vacation, change your way of life, or become ill. Nausea and vomiting accompany certain types of illnesses; clear liquids containing regular sugar are often recommended during these times, since they are absorbed by the body with greater ease, and the energy from the calories helps give you the strength to get well.

You may have difficulty in adjusting to the fact that you have diabetes mellitus. Home management guides you in learning how to handle this adjustment. Perhaps you don't feel like caring for yourself or you are having trouble getting your family's support. You will receive ideas and suggestions on how to speak with your family; on finding ways to be appropriately assertive; and on finding and using resources to assist you during this period and other times of adjustment.

Learning about the complications of the disease is not meant to upset you but to assist you in making appropriate decisions. If you see that you have an infected toe, get to your health professional so that he or she can assist you in getting your blood-glucose levels as normal as possible, get the toe treated right away, and ensure that you are eating correctly. Taking good care of yourself will most likely mean that the toe will heal faster. The information you receive will assist you in making more appropriate choices rather than thinking, "If I'm going to get a complication of diabetes, why try to do anything?"

Undergraduate Self-Management

This level of self-management involves decision making based on choices you would find useful once or twice a week based on blood-glucose levels taken four times a day a minimum of three days a week.

In the Pattern Approach, you would make the change before the time of the problem after assessing the blood-glucose patterns obtained by checking blood sugars four or more times a day for approximately three to five days. For instance, if blood-glucose levels were elevated before suppertime, you would increase the morning intermediate-acting insulin or the short-acting or rapid-acting insulin administered before lunch or decrease or omit a snack or increase the activity level during the interim. If the elevation was before bedtime, you would consider increasing the short-acting or rapid-acting insulin or decreasing the food intake or planning to exercise after supper.

The directions of our program state that you would try this three times with a three-day hold for each time a new regimen is tried. If you still did not see what you expected, you would call your health professional and get direction as to the next regimen to consider. These boundaries of trials would hold true for the graduate level of self-management, too.

Graduate Self-Management

In this level of management, you would become so familiar with your responses to insulin in relation to types and amount of food eaten and the activity level involved that you would be able to predict how much insulin you would need prior to the meal to keep your blood-glucose levels normal or nearly so after the meal. This would require the taking and monitoring of blood-glucose levels before and one to two hours after meals in relation to a variety of food combinations or individually chosen foods and food amounts.

Choosing an Education Program

How can you identify a quality education program? In the past, this was quite a problem. Today this is no longer a problem because a program can be considered high quality if it has passed the rigors of Self-Recognition (a process developed by the American Diabetes Association, in cooperation with the National Diabetes Advisory Board). This recognition means not only that the staff is recognized as being "acceptable" but also that the program's plan, content, and evaluation process are considered to be within certain specific guidelines.

In such a program, one or more of the staff members are certified diabetes educators (CDEs). A CDE has taken the national board examination and has met the qualifications developed by the American Association of Diabetes Educators. The person's experience must include 1,000 hours of actual practice over at least a two-year period in the field of diabetes education, plus a passing score on a written examination. It does not, of course, mean that this person is perfect! It does mean that he or she has a basic knowledge about diabetes, about how to educate another person, and about how to evaluate the process of patient education to see whether success has been achieved.

If your local program and staff members have not yet achieved certification, encourage them to do so. They may already be in the process of applying for recognition and certification. The following topics must be included for a program to be considered for recognition:

- Diabetes disease process
- Nutritional management
- Physical activity
- Medications
- Monitoring
- Acute complications
- Chronic complications
- Goal setting/problem solving
- Psychosocial adjustment
- Preconception/conception care

It is possible that your program has a physician provider, an individual who has met the American Diabetes Association requirements in the provider-recognition program; and an advanced diabetes practitioner (nurse, dietitian, or pharmacist) who has been working for five or more years, has 5,000 hours of experience in the diabetes field, and has passed the national diabetes certification examination given by the American Nurses Certification Corporation (ANCC), that is, board certified in advanced diabetes management (BC-ADM).

The American Association of Diabetes Educators can tell you how to get in touch with a certified diabetes educator. The American Diabetes Association also has a listing of physician providers who have completed and passed the criteria set forth by that organization's leadership. These are physicians who might be endocrinologists, internists, family physicians, or pediatricians who have chosen to specialize in this field.

How Can Education Help You?

Education can help you recognize whether you are receiving up-to-date treatment. It can assist you in making choices on a daily basis. It will help you to know when you should call your health professional and when it isn't necessary to call. Education will help you feel more confident in your self-care practices. Because you will know where your local and national resources are, if you have a question or need a service you will not need to waste valuable time searching for a resource.

Education can also help your family and friends. They, too, have some adjusting to do. If they do not adjust, you may feel rejected or not supported in the manner that might be more beneficial. If your family and friends learn about diabetes, they will not feel as if they have to "walk on eggshells" when they are around you. They will not have to ask you if you can do this or that or if you can eat this or that. It is true that because they will know what you should do, they may use that information in a nagging way. But if they have truly listened in the classroom and group settings, they will know that nagging is not the thing to do. They will know how best to support you in your endeavor to keep yourself healthy. In fact, they may become healthier as they follow the instructions for the type of health care program that you are requested to follow. Also, two heads are better than one: When a question arises, you can check with a family member to see whether he or she understood the information given in class in the same way you did.

Most important, you should recognize that you are not alone and that there are many people interested in your welfare. A good education regarding your diabetes is vital to you and your family. Demand it, and use it.

5

How Should You Eat?

Meal planning involves learning how to choose foods and eating the appropriate amounts. The so-called diabetic diet is no different from the diet that all people ought to be eating. It includes plenty of fruits and vegetables; lean meat, chicken, and fish; whole-grain breads and cereals; and low-fat dairy products. The recommended proportions are 30 percent or less fat, 12 to 20 percent protein, and the rest in carbohydrates called simple sugars and complex carbohydrates, such as cereals, fruits, and vegetables. (See Appendix A for help in evaluating your own dietary intake.)

Two major considerations in restricting simple sugars—such as table sugar, honey, and molasses—are:

1. A timing factor: With the development of analogue insulins (also called *designer insulins* because they can be made to respond in a shorter or longer period of time just by changing the sequence of some of the amino acids), it is easier to "cover" the rapidly rising blood sugar caused by the more concentrated sweets.
2. "Empty calories": These foods contain very little, if any, nutritional value.

Basic Eating Guidelines

Much of our life is spent planning what to eat, preparing food, and eating food. In order for the food to be absorbed, it must be broken into tiny particles. The simpler the food item, the easier it is to absorb. In fact, a few teaspoons of honey given by mouth is absorbed almost as fast as glucose injected in a vein. These tiny particles may be completely changed to glucose and have little, if any, nutritional value, or they may contain varying amounts of protein, fat, vitamins, and minerals. Whatever the "food particle," the basic form of storage is glucose.

The three basic food sources are carbohydrates for energy; protein for cellular growth and repair; and fat for heat and an alternative source of energy. (See Figure 5.1 for the complete Food Guide Pyramid.) All of these food sources can, to a certain extent, be changed into the carbohydrate glucose, but none of the food sources, including carbohydrates, can be changed into protein. Carbohydrates may be stored as fats (triglycerides), but fats may not be stored as carbohydrates unless they are broken down into parts that include some glucose.

It is recommended that people with diabetes eat a well-balanced diet of nourishing foods that have appropriate nutrients rather than simple sugars having few, if any, important nutrients. Eating the designated portions of these foods at appropriate times will help control the blood-sugar level and maintain the body weight proportionate to the height of the person. Since fat contains a concentrated source of calories, it should be eaten in very limited quantities. To help maintain weight or lose it, if necessary, food intake should be distributed throughout the day into frequent small meals and snacks. This is often patterned into three meals and zero to one or more snacks. The slowest-absorbing food group, protein, should also be distributed appropriately throughout the day to sustain blood-glucose levels. To aid in digestion and the proper rate of food absorption, a high fiber content is recommended. High-fiber foods include whole-grain breads and cereals, fruits, and vegetables.

The person who has diabetes should have a food intake made up of nutritious foods containing the needed vitamins and minerals, carbohydrates, proteins, and fats, accompanied by adequate water intake. (See Appendix B for Recommended Dietary Allowances.)

Figure 5.1 Food Guide Pyramid

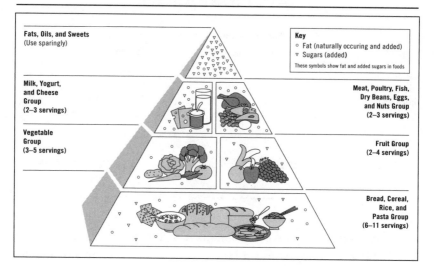

Carbohydrates

Carbohydrates are the body's source of fuel, giving the body energy to be active and to carry on its daily metabolic activities. Carbohydrates contain 4 calories per gram of weight. Simple carbohydrates are found in simple sugars, such as table sugar, honey, corn syrup, sorghum, date sugar, molasses, brown sugar, powdered sugar, turbinado sugar, and any substance that ends in *ose* (for example, glucose and fructose).

Complex carbohydrates are cereals, breads, pastas, and vegetables. Fruit contains both simple and complex carbohydrates. Simple carbohydrates are digested rapidly; complex carbohydrates are digested more slowly.

Fats

Fat contains a more concentrated source of calories (with 9 calories per gram) than do carbohydrates or protein. Fats carry vitamins and important or essential fatty acids. Examples of fatty foods include butter and margarine, cream, salad dressings, oils, and lard. Some foods, such as avocados, olives, and certain nuts, contain large amounts of fat.

Table 5.1 Types of Dietary Fat

Type of Fat	Appearance at Room Temperature	Example
Saturated	Solid	Butter, lard
Monounsaturated	Liquid	Olive oil
Polyunsaturated	Liquid	Corn oil, safflower oil
Cholesterol	Solid	Food derived from animals
(liquid when heated)		
Triglycerides*		

*Triglycerides, as their name implies, are made up of three fatty acids bound together by a carbohydrate, sugar alcohol (glycerol).

There are five terms in the language of fat that you should know (see Table 5.1). The American Heart Association recommends the use of monounsaturated fats in controlling heart disease.

Cholesterol is a fatlike alcohol found in animal fats and oils. Most of it is developed in the liver, but it can also be absorbed from the diet. Cholesterol is blamed for much of the heart disease in our culture. Research indicates that it is one of cholesterol's fats—low-density lipoprotein cholesterol (LDL)—that is one of the main culprits. High-density lipoprotein (HDL) cholesterol is the "good guy." Triglyceride in the body is affected by the cholesterol, glucose, and saturated fat in the diet. When the blood sugar is lowered, the triglyceride level is usually lowered, too.

Proteins

Proteins have four calories per gram and are the most slowly absorbed foods. Until the early 1980s, fats were considered to be the slowest-absorbing of the three food groups. Research from a university on the east coast determined otherwise. Proteins have a greater than 50 percent capability of being changed into glucose. While fats must be changed into ketone bodies before being used as an energy source, proteins need only to be changed into glucose.

All animal sources contain protein. This includes dairy products, meats, and fish. Vegetable plant sources contain protein, but in varying amounts. Grains also contain protein. The recommended amount for adults is 12 to 15 percent of the diet, and for children 15 to 20 percent.

Other Nutrients

Other nutrients are also important in meeting the needs of the human body. Nutrients are found both in minerals (such as iron and calcium) and in vitamins (as in A, B_1, B_2, B_3, C, D, and so forth). Along with the three food groups, nutrients are needed as an energy source and are used for growth and repair of body tissue. Although there are roughly fifty or more nutrients needed for daily growth and development, only the major vitamins and minerals are discussed here.

Iron is the carrier of oxygen to body tissues. Anemia is prevented through adequate iron in the diet. Calcium is used for building strong bones and teeth; it is also used in muscle contraction and relaxation and in the proper functioning of the nerves. Vitamin A is known for its role in promoting good vision. Its lesser but still important role is in keeping the skin and mucous membranes in good condition.

Vitamin B_1 aids in digestion and in muscle and nerve function. B_2 helps in promoting healthy skin and mucous membranes and general vitality. B_3 aids in digestion and keeps the nerves and skin in good condition. Vitamin C has many more roles than was thought earlier. It helps not only in the healing processes but also in maintaining healthy gums, bones, tissues, blood, and blood vessels. Vitamin D assists in the utilization of calcium and in the maintenance of healthy bones.

Baseline Meal Planning

Meal plans are meant to help you rather than to be an obstacle. They should be individualized to meet your particular needs, wants, and lifestyle and organized within the bounds of your particular health problem(s). The plan must meet the caloric level of your daily activity unless you are overweight, in which case you need to decrease your caloric intake in relation to the calories you burn in daily activity (with a weight-loss goal of from one-half to two pounds per week).

The three most important things to keep in mind are as follows:

1. Be sure that you are getting the nutrition you need to meet your energy demands.
2. The food should be distributed throughout the day so that the body is not overwhelmed at any one time.
3. The food pattern and amounts eaten should be consistent, unless a greater or lesser energy use requires a greater or lesser amount of food intake.

The purpose of a meal plan is to help you achieve these important goals. A meal plan may be developed using a variety of methods. To figure out the ideal body weight for a female, take the height (for example, 5'4") and give 100 pounds for the first five feet and five pounds for each inch above five feet. That would be $100 + (4 \times 5)$, for an ideal body weight of 120 pounds for a medium-boned female, plus or minus 10 percent to allow for differences in bone structure (that is, large boned or small boned). For males, 106 pounds are given for the first five feet of height, and six pounds for each inch above five feet. For a male who is 5'11" tall, the calculation would be $106 + (11 \times 6) = 172$ pounds, plus or minus 10 percent to account for bone structure.

The average recommended dietary intake is 10 to 15 calories per pound (20 to 30 calories per kilogram), depending on whether you are male or female and active or inactive. A pregnant woman requires up to 17 calories per pound (39 calories/kg), especially during the last trimester; nursing mothers also require this amount and usually more. An infant needs roughly 55 calories per pound, and a school-age child needs 30 or more calories per pound.

Infants and small children need their calories to be distributed throughout the day in a pattern of three meals and one to three between-meal snacks. Children, especially, thrive on three meals and three snacks. Because their stomachs are too small to hold large quantities of food at mealtimes and their ability to store glucose is limited because of their size, some food intake every two or three hours is appropriate. As they grow, children need an increase in caloric intake to meet their needs. This can be figured scientifically with a chart or mathematical calculation. It can also be done by noting when the child is consistently eating more than the baseline meal plan that was calculated in the office or hospital, and then increasing the total meal plan by that extra number of calories (usually in increments of 100 or 200 calories).

The goal of any meal plan is to meet caloric and nutritional requirements with high-fiber, low-fat foods, with few or no concentrated sweets. The meal plan should be altered for changes in growth, activity level, and lifestyle.

The major approaches to meal planning are carbohydrate counting, the exchange lists (composed of six food groups—see Appendix C), calorie points (see Appendixes D and E), and the "Idaho Plate Method."

Carbohydrate counting is a method of dietary control for people who have diabetes. This system of diet control was devised by the Diabetes Control and Complications Study (DCCT) to provide better dietary guidelines for persons undergoing intensive diabetes management (the standard exchange list did not work well in this study for intensive management).

Carbohydrate counting means that a person is requested to eat a certain number of servings of carbohydrate foods to equal a certain number of grams of carbohydrate. Little restriction is placed on fat and protein other than following the recommended dietary intake of 12 to 15 percent protein, 30 percent or less fat, and the rest in carbohydrates.

Carbohydrate counting is a system of calculating the carbohydrate composition of foods for each meal and then calculating the insulin dose based on so much insulin for a set amount of carbohydrate. The usual formula is one unit of insulin for every 15 grams of carbohydrate, or 60 calories. The system has much to recommend it in precision and as a mathematical method for determining insulin doses. There are several problems to the system, however, that limit its usefulness. The problems are as follows:

1. The system is complex since the patient has to be able to determine the number of carbohydrate points in each piece of food. This can be very difficult, especially for mixed foods such as casseroles and soups. At our diabetes camp, several children up to sixteen years of age have come insisting on carbohydrate counting and claiming the know-how. When tested by having the dietitian cross-check their calculations on the food line, we found that the majority of the kids didn't have a clue.

2. Foods other than carbohydrate are counted as free in the sense that the person can have as much as they want. This can have two important consequences:

- The extra food can result in too much to eat and obesity.
- There can be an underestimation of the insulin need. Protein also requires insulin for its metabolism, and 50 percent or more of it is converted to carbohydrate. This carbohydrate requires insulin but does not enter into the insulin dose calculation. Thus the person may be underinsulinized and in poor diabetes control. Hemoglobin A1c values of the children at camp using carbohydrate counting were on average two points higher than the children using the point system (9.4 percent versus 7.4 percent).

The exchange lists are discussed in detail in the appendixes. They contain six food groupings: starch, meat, vegetable, fruit, milk, and fat. These food groups are distributed throughout the day in predetermined amounts.

The point system was first planned for a non-English-speaking population in Chicago. It can be used to plan for a certain amount of carbohydrate, protein, fat, major vitamins and minerals, cholesterol, sodium, and calories. We use the calorie system where 75 calories equals one point. (It has been used for the carbohydrate [CHO] counting, i.e., 15 grams CHO equals one point). The food is distributed throughout the day in various serving sizes. Some of the more common distributions are noted in Table 5.2.

Therefore, carbohydrate counting is a variation of the point system (CHO = 1 pt; 1 oz P = ½ pt), but in the point system all calories are used to calculate medicine needs. It is also easier to calculate total points or calories than to try to sort out only the carbohydrates. The point calculation is simple and based on everyday food usage—for example, one slice of bread is one point, one glass of skim milk is one point, one ounce of meat or cheese is one point, and so on. The point system is easy to learn and it works well. We use it daily with hundreds of patients with good results.

The "Idaho Plate Method" of meal planning was reported in the literature in 1998. It is useful for people with low reading skills who

Table 5.2 Standard Calorie-Point Distribution

| | | | 3 MEALS AND 3 SNACKS | | | | |
| | Calorie | Breakfast | Morning Snack | Lunch | Afternoon Snack | Evening Meal | Bedtime Snack |
Calories	Points	4/18*	1/18*	5/18*	2/18*	5/18*	1/18*
1,000	13.5	3	1	3.5	1.5	3.5	1
1,200	16	3.5	1	4.5	1.5	4.5	1
1,400	18.5	4	1	5	2	5.5	1
1,600	21.5	5	1	6	2	6	1.5
1,800	24	5.5	1.5	6.5	2.5	6.6	1.5
2,000	26.5	6	1.5	7	3	7	2
2,500	33.5	7.5	2	9	3.5	9.5	2
3,000	40	9	2	11	4.5	11.5	2

*Of total calorie intake

need to lose weight or who have trouble with more structured approaches. Simply put, the plate is divided for breakfast into only one-quarter of optional meat/protein and one-half starch/bread; for lunch and dinner, one-quarter starch/bread, one-quarter meat/protein, and one-half vegetables. One serving on the plate should not touch another. Milk and fruit should be served at each mealtime.

Special Needs

If weight loss is necessary, the meal plan will need to change. It takes the equivalent of just one extra slice of bread per day to result in a pound of weight gain in a month. Weight loss requires following these rules:

1. The intake must be less than the energy output.
2. The food intake must be distributed throughout the day.
3. Food intake should be limited to the daylight hours, and food should not be eaten later than two to three hours before bedtime unless the person is on insulin (in which case, depending on his or her diabetes medication program, there might be a bedtime snack).

4. A vitamin supplement is recommended if the total caloric level is below 1,200 calories per day. (Any plan below this level will have difficulty meeting the recommended daily requirements of vitamins and minerals.)

5. Liquid-protein diets are recommended only for the greatly overweight person, and any person using liquid-protein products should be closely monitored by a physician.

6. An exercise program must be carried out on a daily or every-other-day basis.

Elevation in cholesterol or triglycerides requires a careful monitoring and restriction of fat intake (and, especially for triglycerides, restriction of alcohol intake). Again, exercise is helpful for both of these conditions. For triglyceride problems, the normalization of blood-glucose levels is helpful. If hyperlipidemia (high fat content in the blood) is a genetic rather than a dietary problem, the health professional will prescribe appropriate medication dosages to assist in normalizing the cholesterol and/or triglyceride levels.

Hypertension (high blood pressure) may require a decrease in salt intake. This problem may be due to kidney disease (nephropathy) or to other factors, such as age and weight. If you have complications from your diabetes, hypertension may aggravate them. In any case, normalizing your blood pressure is accomplished by taking the medication prescribed by your health professional and eating nutritiously, both in amounts and choices. Keep the saltshaker off the table. Refrain from eating salty foods such as hot dogs, TV dinners, most canned soups, and potato chips. Although salt substitutes may be used, fresh foods usually contain enough sodium chloride (table salt) for bodily needs.

Preventing hypoglycemia means that you need to carry some form of simple sugar or food with you at all times. Foods to carry might be dried fruits or packets of crackers. Granola bars or small cans of juice would also be helpful to have on hand. These foods could be used when there is an unexpected increase in activity level, for planned extra activity, or when low blood-glucose levels need treatment (that is, when blood sugar is higher than 40 mg/dl [2.2 mmol]). Below that level, simple sugar is needed.

Food intake during illness varies. If someone is experiencing nausea, with or without vomiting, clear liquids will be needed. Some health professionals recommend that the clear liquids not contain any sugar until the blood-glucose levels are below 300 mg/dl (17 mmol). Others say that calories are still needed for the energy required to combat the illness, with insulin supplements given to compensate for the elevation in blood-glucose levels. Almost all health professionals agree that during an illness accompanied by nausea, vomiting, and diarrhea, a patient with blood-glucose levels in the 200 mg/dl (11.1 mmol) range or lower requires clear, sugar-containing liquids for twenty-four to forty-eight hours. The person may then progress to eating crackers and dry toast. If the crackers and toast are tolerated, soups and other light foods may be tried.

If activity level decreases, then fewer total calories are needed. For illness, the usual recommendation is to consume 20 percent fewer total calories than you usually need on an active day. This amount would be increased when activity returns to its usual level. The principles to remember are as follows:

1. Fewer calories are needed when the body is at rest.
2. Simpler foods are easier to digest.
3. Fluid intake (noncaloric or low-calorie beverages) should be encouraged unless nausea, vomiting, and diarrhea are present. If these are present or if blood sugars fall to 300 mg/dl (16.6 mmol) or less, then sugar-containing fluids will help prevent ketogenesis (using ketones for energy rather than glucose).
4. If you are on a weight loss program, plan to lose only one-half to one pound per week if you are a woman and one to two pounds per week if you are a man (the faster it comes off, the faster it goes back on).
5. *If in doubt, contact your health professional.*

New diet options are always appearing. Some have a higher protein content. It is true that you don't feel as hungry and your blood sugars will fluctuate less (fewer ups and downs) with a high-protein diet, but you need to have well-functioning kidneys and be able to drink more than eight glasses of water each day (to prevent an "illness" that can result from large amounts of protein in the blood). The liquid high-protein diets have been documented to "wash" calcium out of the system. Also, be aware that if you choose to go on such a diet your health should be monitored by a health professional.

Every change in health level or activity level needs individual attention at the time of the change. If you have not been educated to make the appropriate changes yourself, contact your health professional for advice.

6

What About Medications?

People who have diabetes mellitus need one or more types of medication to control their blood sugar unless they are able to control their blood-glucose levels with lifestyle changes. One type of medication assists in the use of insulin (part of the action of the sufonylureas and thiazolidinediones [TZDs]) and availability of insulin (sulfonylureas; meglitinides—benzoic-acid based or a derivative of the amino acid D-phenylalanine). Another type of medication replaces the body's insulin when the body is no longer able to make insulin, while other types of medication block the formation of new glucose in the liver (biguanides—decrease hepatic glucose production) or block the absorption of carbohydrates from the intestine (alpha glucosidase inhibitors). The choice(s) depends on the body's needs in relation to the type of diabetes with which he person has been diagnosed.

For people with Type 2 diabetes, if the average blood-glucose levels are greater than 150 mg/dl (8.3 mmol), then an oral hypoglycemic agent is needed. Unless what is going on in your body suggests otherwise (e.g., you are unable or unwilling to lose weight, or your blood sugar is high in spite of weight loss), you will need one or eventually two or more types of oral diabetes medication (see Table 6.1).

If the oral agent combinations are used at the maximum dosage level and are still not effective (that is, they are unable to lower after-meal blood sugars to below 180 mg/dl [10 mmol]), then insulin is needed (usually starting with a bedtime dose). In many cases, insulin and oral agents are combined.

Oral Diabetes Agents

Oral diabetes agents are not insulin "pills" but powdered, compressed medications that control the level of glucose in the body by a variety of ways. These medications appear to affect the insulin-making ability of the beta cells of the pancreas, stimulate the formation of receptor sites on the cells, stimulate the insulin-binding action at the receptor sites, or aid in correcting some postreceptor defects inside the cells, or a combination of these. Other medications affect the production of glucose by the liver or keep the intestine from absorbing carbohydrates.

You must have some insulin-making ability to be able to respond to an oral diabetes agent. If your body is not making enough insulin or the cells in your body are not able to correctly use the insulin you are making, and if simple control of dietary intake (or getting your body weight closer to a healthy level) is not effective, you probably need an oral agent to help control your blood-glucose levels. If one or a combination of agents does not work for you, then another choice of medication is made or additional medication is needed.

Many people think that if they are taking oral agents they do not need to watch their dietary intake. This is not true. For the healthiest responses, you should still make nutritious choices, space out the meals, and include one or more snacks each day while also following the other parts of your self-care program. It is also important to check your blood-glucose levels to be sure that the medication is working to meet the goal of premeal blood-glucose levels of between 70 to 110 mg/dl (3.8 to 6.1 mmol) and two-hour postmeal (postprandial) levels of less than 150 mg/dl (8.3 mmol), or at least less than 180 mg/dl (10 mmol), and an overall goal of less than 7 percent for the HbA1c (hemoglobin A1c).

You must also be knowledgeable about the side effects of oral agents. These are hypoglycemia (low blood sugar), nausea, and vomiting. Yellowing of the skin (jaundice) and skin rashes have also been reported. Except for hypoglycemia, these side effects occur in fewer than 1 percent of people taking these medications. Metformins, thiazolidinediones, and alpha glucosidase inhibitors will not cause hypoglycemia when used alone but may do so when used with other agents.

Metformins, thiazolidinediones, and alpha glucosidase inhibitors do not have hypoglycemia as a side effect but do have other side effects. Metformins may cause an upset of the intestinal tract, especially diar-

Table 6.1 Oral Diabetes Agents

Action	Generic Name	Trade Name
Rapid and Short Acting (2 to 4 ×/day)	Tolbutamide (sulfonylurea)	Orinase
	Repaglinide (benzoic-acid based)	Prandin
	Nateglinide (D-phenylalanine derivative)	Starlix
Intermediate Acting (1 to 2 ×/day) (sulfonylureas)	Acetohexamide	Dymelor
	Tolazamide	Tolinase
	Glyburide	Micronase, DiaBeta
	Glyburide Micronized	Glynase Prestab
	Glipizide	Glucotrol, Glucotrol XL
	Glimepiride	Amaryl
Long Acting (1 ×/day) (sulfonylureas)	Clorpropamide	Diabinase
Insulin-Sensitizing Agents (thiazolidinediones)	Pioglitazone	Actos (1 to 2 ×/day)
	Rosiglitazone	Avandia
Hepatic Glucose Blockers (biguanides)	Metformin	Glucophage Glucophage XR (extended release)
Combined Agents (biguanides/sulfonylureas)	Glyburide/Metformin	Glucovance
	Metformin/Glipizide	Metaglip
(thiazolidinediones/biguanides)	Rosiglitazone/Metformin	Avandamet
Alpha Glucosidase Inhibitors	Acarbose	Precose
	Miglitol	Glyset

rhea. This is usually seen only at the start of treatment and usually goes away in one to two weeks. This problem can be minimized if the metformin is started at low doses and given with food. A metal taste in the mouth has also been reported.

Thiazolidinediones may result in some elevation in liver enzymes called transaminases (now rarely seen). These enzymes should be monitored every two months for the first year and then at each regular office visit. Ankle edema has also been noted.

Alpha glucosidase inhibitors may stimulate the occurrence of increased intestinal gas and subsequent bloating.

You need to be familiar with the interaction of your diabetes medication(s) with any other medications you might be taking. Drinking alcohol while you are taking chlorpropamide may result in an antabuse type of reaction (flushing of the skin, nausea, and vomiting). With the first-generation oral hypoglycemic agents, taking another drug the same day may cause either the drug or the oral agents to work more or less effectively (by "bumping" medications off their binding sites on the receptors). Drugs that may interact with these oral agents include anticoagulants, birth control pills, diuretics, steroids, and Dilantin (which raise the blood sugar), as well as some drugs that lower blood sugar, including aspirin and some medicines used to treat high blood pressure (such as Inderal). These interactions do not seem to occur with second-generation sulfonlyureas agents.

The only oral agent presently prescribed for children with Type 2 diabetes is metformin. You may need to stop an oral agent and have it replaced by insulin for a period of time if you are pregnant, nursing, ill, or having surgery.

You also need to be familiar with the time action of the oral hypoglycemic agents you are taking. Knowing this allows you to either predict or determine the potential for hypoglycemic episodes.

Rapid- and Short-Acting Agents

One short-acting oral agent is called tolbutamide (the generic name) or Orinase (the brand name). If your physician writes the generic name on the prescription, you can often receive the product at its lowest cost (available through the Barr, Danberry, Lederle, and Zenith companies). Orinase is available in 500-mg tablets from the Pharmacia drug company. It starts working in one hour and is half used in about 5.6 hours; the total time it works in the body is approximately six to twelve hours. The recommended dosage is usually no more than 2 g (or four 500-mg tablets) per day. The maximum dose is 3 g per day (seldom used).

Repaglinide (Prandin), a benzoic acid derivative, is a rapid-acting oral agent produced by Novo-Nordisk. This medication is from a different class of drugs (meglitinides) that can be used in people allergic to the other oral drugs, but it works in a similar though not exactly the same way as the sulfonylureas. It acts more quickly than the other drugs so it is given right before meals. It keeps the after-meal blood sugar down and then is gone from the body rather quickly, so it doesn't linger and cause low blood sugars later. It is very effective but has the inconvenience of having to be taken three to four times a day. It has the convenience of very few side effects and little hypoglycemia. It is also convenient in that a dose can be skipped if a meal is skipped. The sulfonylureas last longer and may cause hypoglycemia if a meal is missed, but not so with this rapid-acting drug. Thus there is more schedule flexibility with this drug. The doses of Prandin range from 1 to 4 mg three times a day with meals to 4 mg with each meal and before a bedtime snack.

Nateglinide (Starlix) is also of the meglitinide classification. It is produced by Novartis. Nateglinide is usually administered in 120-mg tablets, one tablet before each meal. It is also available in a 60-mg size and is recommended when initially combined with a metformin. Nateglinide is a derivative of the amino acid D-phenylalanine. This medication acts directly on the pancreatic beta cell, so it is taken just before a meal in order to control the after-meal hyperglycemia.

Intermediate-Acting Agents

The intermediate-acting oral agents are acetohexamide (Dymelor by Lilly) and tolazamide (Tolinase by Pharmacia) from the first generation, and glipizide (Glucotrol, Glucotrol XL by Pfizer), glimepiride (Amaryl by Aventis), and glyburide (Micronase by Pharmacia, DiaBeta by Aventis, and Glynase Prestab by Pharmacia) from the second generation (see Table 6.1). The first-generation pills were tested and put on the market in the 1950s and 1960s. The second-generation pills were tested in the United States and put on the market in the 1970s and 1980s.

Acetohexamide (Dymelor) comes in 250-mg and 500-mg tablets. Dymelor is usually administered (500-mg to 750-mg) once a day or in divided doses. This medication starts working in about one hour, and over half of its usefulness occurs within five hours. It stays in the body for approximately ten to fourteen hours. The maximum dosage recommended is 1.5 g per day (six 250-mg tablets or three 500-mg tablets). If you have problems with improper functioning of your kidneys, this medication would not be recommended. It is available in the generic form, which costs less than the seldom-used brand-name drug.

Tolazamide (Tolinase) is an oral agent that is absorbed more slowly (its onset is four to six hours). If you have a tendency to absorb food slowly, then this oral agent might be recommended for you. It comes in 100-mg, 250-mg, and 500-mg tablets and is made by Pfizer (Pharmacia). Half of the usefulness of this medication occurs in your body within approximately seven hours. The maximum recommended dosage is 1 g per day (ten 100-mg tablets, four 250-mg tablets, or two 500-mg tablets). This product is also available as a generic through the Barr, Danbury, Lederle, and Zenith drug companies, but is rarely used.

Glyburide, the generic form, is also available as a brand-name product through the Pharmacia company (Micronase and Glynase Prestab) and the Aventis company (DiaBeta). The tablet sizes are 1.25 mg, 2.5 mg, and 5 mg. The maximum dose recommended is 20 mg per day. Glynase is a more bioactive drug than the others (i.e., it is easily absorbed so it is slightly better). It is available in both the generic form and the Prestab form (easily breakable), given as 3-mg and 6-mg tablets once or twice a day (top dose is 12 mg per day). These tablets are easily broken into two pieces. As with any other intermediate-acting oral agent, the daily dosage is usually divided (into before breakfast and before supper doses) when 10 mg or more of medication is needed. The onset is 1.5 hours, and the total duration is around twenty-four hours. Half of the medication's usefulness may occur in from 3.2 hours, for part of its chemical action, to ten hours. Half of this medication is excreted in the urine and the other half through the bile in the liver, but caution is still encouraged for use in the elderly.

Glipizide (Glucotrol; Glucotrol XL, a sustained release tablet) is marketed by Pfizer in a 5-mg and 10-mg tablet. It is also available in the generic form. The half-life of this medication is 3.5 to six hours. It may remain in the body for anywhere from twelve to sixteen hours. It is recommended that a total of no more than 40 mg of Glucotrol or no more than 20 mg of Glucotrol XL be taken in a single day. Although Glucotrol XL may be taken with a meal, it is recommended that regular Glucotrol be taken on an empty stomach (that is, about thirty minutes before a meal) to achieve the best level of activity. If more than 15 mg of Glucotrol is needed, the dose should be divided. Although both of these medications are changed to an inactive form in the liver, caution is highly recommended if liver disease is present, especially in the elderly.

Glimepiride (Amaryl by Aventis) is also a sulfonylurea oral hypo-glycemic agent. This drug has the advantage of being insulin sparing. Glimepiride works by making the available insulin more effective by its effects on muscle and fat cells and on the liver. The drug is taken once a day in 1-, 2-, and 4-mg tablet sizes. The starting dose is 1 mg per day. The dose can be increased every two to four weeks if the full ther-apeutic effect is not achieved. The maximum dose is 8 mg per day.

Antihyperglycemic Agents

Metformin (Glucophage; Glucophage XR produced by Bristol-Myers Squibb) affects the body in several ways: 20 percent of its action increases the body's sensitivity to insulin, increasing the muscles' abil-ity to use insulin; 80 percent of its action prevents glucose production in the liver. Metformin has been found to reduce levels of triglycerides and other fats such as LDL ("bad") cholesterol in the blood, and may decrease the absorption of glucose from the intestine. All of these effects usually result in lower blood sugar. Side effects may include loss of appetite, a metal taste in the mouth, nausea, and diarrhea; however, metformin does not promote weight gain. Metformin is available in 500-mg, 850-mg, and 1,000-mg tablets, with a maximum dosage of 2,550 mg per day. Contraindications for metformin include patients with Type 1 diabetes; those at risk for cardiovascular disease; those with kidney or liver disease; those with serum creatinine levels greater than 1.4 for men and 1.5 for women; those who use alcohol excessively; and children and pregnant women. The use of metformin with any of these conditions can result in serious and potentially fatal side effects such as lacticacidosis (lactic acid or organic acid buildup in muscle cells and bloodstream). Metformin can be used in combination with such oral hypoglycemic agents as acarbose, naglitinide, rosiglitizone, nateglinide, or insulin. It is presently available combined with glyburide in a pill called Glucovance or with rosiglitazone called Avandamet.

Alpha glucosidase inhibitors include acarbose (Precose by Bayer) and miglitol (Glyset by Pharmacia). They work in the small intestine to slow the breakdown of carbohydrates, particularly complex carbo-hydrates. Acarbose and miglitol slow down the natural breakdown of starches, dextrins, maltose, and sucrose to absorbable monosac-charides. They are therefore most effective for people who have high glucose levels after eating. Acarbose and miglitol are taken just before meals, or with the first bite of each meal. Doses begin with one 25-mg dose with the first bite of a meal. Tablets for dosing are 50 mg three times a day (or before each meal) if the person weighs less than 130 pounds (60 kg)or 100 mg three times a day (or before each meal) if the person weighs 130 pounds (60 kg) or more. Side effects include abdominal pain, diarrhea, and flatulence. Neither acarbose nor miglitol are to be used with patients who have inflammatory bowel disease, colonic ulceration, or partial intestinal obstruction. They can be used alone or in combination with any of the other drugs and/or insulins.

Thiazolidinediones include pioglitazone (Actos by Takeda) and rosiglitazone (Avandia by GlaxoSmithKline). They are oral antihyperglycemic agents that act to decrease insulin resistance (80 percent of their activity; 20 percent of their activity is effective in blocking hepatic glucose production). Their complete action is unknown, but they are thought to stimulate the production of a protein involved in the transport of glucose in the blood through the cell membrane to the interior of the cell. It takes two to six weeks for the medicine to have much effect on blood-glucose levels and may take as long as twelve weeks for it to have its full effect. The medicine is taken with food to enhance its absorption. It can be taken with any meal but needs to be taken only once a day. It is absorbed in two to three hours. If it is missed at the usual meal, it may be taken at the next meal. If it is missed on one day, it should not be doubled the next day. More than 85 percent of the medicine's waste products are removed through the intestinal tract, and only a little over 3 percent are released through the urine. Thiazolidinediones are not recommended for pregnant or breast-feeding women or people with severe heart disease.

Thiazolidinediones may be used alone, with other oral agents, or with insulin. A person would start with 15 to 30 mg once daily for rosiglitazone or 2 to 4 mg once daily for pioglitazone, usually with a meal. After two to four weeks, the dose may, if needed, be increased to a maximum of 45 mg once a day for rosiglitazone or 8 mg in a single or divided dose for pioglitazone. If a person with Type 2 diabetes is already on insulin, it is recommended that after a thiazolidinedione is started, insulin may be decreased by 10 to 25 percent or more when fasting blood sugars are less than 120 mg/dl (6.6 mmol). One value of this class of drug is that it is remarkably free of side effects, even at maximal doses, though ankle edema is a possibility. Another benefit is the effect on lipids or fats in the blood (i.e., lower type of low-density lipoprotein), the fat associated with a higher risk of heart attack.

If you are to start on a thiazolidinedione (Actos or Avandia), be sure your physician checks your liver function via laboratory work before you take the medication, again every two months for the first year, and then at every regular doctor visit (i.e., every three to four months). If this is done, there is little or no danger from these drugs. Actos and Avandia are highly effective drugs that have vastly improved diabetes control in thousands of patients.

Combination Medications

As of this writing, there are three combined medicines available in the United States (see Table 6.1): Glucovance (glyburide and metformin), Metaglip (metformin and glipizide), and Avandamet (rosiglitazone and metformin). Each of these mixtures, even in lower doses, appears to have a greater effect in decreasing blood glucose levels than when used individually.

General Recommendations

Oral hypoglycemic and antihyperglycemic agents have an important place in the medical management of diabetes. They can be used alone or in combination with each other and/or with insulin. When the blood sugar is no longer controlled by the maximum recommended amount of an oral medication, there is no other recourse than to administer insulin. (Note: Taking more of an oral agent than what is recommended could make you quite sick.)

Insulin

Before insulin was discovered, a child who had diabetes could expect to live only about two years from the time of diagnosis. Insulin was first chemically removed from the pancreas of animals, but now some form of biological engineering using recombinant-DNA technology makes human insulin. Using animal-derived insulin (highly purified pork or

beef or a pork/beef mix) is now almost a thing of the past. Eli Lilly &
Co. does fill special orders for purified pork insulin as it does have a
longer duration of action.

Like oral hypoglycemic agents, insulin is available in rapid-acting,
short-acting, intermediate-acting, and long-acting forms (see Table 6.2,
page 62). Lente (L) is a premixed, crystalline, intermediate-acting insulin.
The long-acting form, ultralente (U), contains a smaller number of crystals, but they are larger in size. Lente insulin is a mixture of the two types
(30 percent semilente—no longer available as a separate insulin—and 70
percent ultralente), but because of the slower onset of the lente insulin,
Lente is at times mixed with short-acting regular or a rapid-acting insulin
to get a quicker early action along with the more prolonged action.

When a protein called protamine is attached to a short-acting
insulin, it becomes NPH (neutral protamine hagedorn [N]), an intermediate-acting insulin. In the newer insulin, called designer or "tailored"
insulin, some of the proteins in the insulin chain will have their sequence
changed. This will result in a change in the time action of insulin. If a
person is allergic to the type of protein found in NPH, lente is a good
substitute. The major side effects that can occur when taking insulin
injections are as follows:

- Low blood sugar/hypoglycemia (also called insulin reaction or
  insulin shock)
- Hypertrophy (an enlarged area that results from receiving the
  shot in the same place for too long)
- Atrophy (a sunken area, as a response to the insulin and its
  diluting agent; has been observed less frequently with the
  advent of human insulin)
- A rash at the site of the injection or a rash all over the body

These and other side effects are seldom noted with the use of human or
designer insulins.

In the United States, insulin is available in a concentration of 100
units per 1 cc, called U100. For special purposes, such as research, U500
(Eli Lilly & Co.) and U400 (Aventis Corporation) are available. Most
other countries are currently in the process of converting their available
insulin into the U100 form. (Note: Some U40 or U80 insulin may be
available in other parts of the world.)

If a child or adult is extremely sensitive to insulin changes, then the insulin may be diluted to U50 (a 1:1 dilution) or U25 (a 1:3 dilution—one part insulin with three parts diluting fluid). This allows changes in the insulin dosage to be made in one-quarter to one-half unit changes rather than one-unit changes. The syringes, such as the fifty-unit syringe (or thirty-unit syringe), allow the careful measuring of single unit change. Therefore, diluting insulin may not be needed except for infants.

Your program should be based on your lifestyle and the energy needed to maintain these activities. Diabetes medication, including insulin, should then be designated at the dosage levels that best keep the blood-glucose levels as normal as possible without causing significant insulin reactions. Therefore, knowing the time action of your diabetes-related medication is very important. Consider the pharmacodynamic action of the medication (therapeutic or the effective action of the medication) over the pharmacokinetic action of the medication insulin. The pharmacokinetic action (also called the pharmacologic action) of insulin is the response of the body to the insulin from the time it enters the body until it is no longer measurable in the body. The therapeutic (effective) duration of action of the insulin is the time a certain amount of insulin will keep your blood-sugar level within the normal range (see Table 3.1, page 22). The former is important to scientists but, although shorter in time action, is more important to the person taking the medication. If you eat more or less than you planned, recognize that hyper- or hypoglycemia may follow if your food intake is not counterbalanced by more or less activity or exercise.

Three companies—Eli Lilly & Co., Novo-Nordisk Pharmaceuticals, and Aventis—are currently producing insulin in the United States. Wal-Mart is now distributing insulin (Reli-on, Novolin-R, Novolin-N, and Novolin 70/30) produced by Novo-Nordisk. These companies, as well as other professionals in the field, are recognizing that there is seldom a case when one dose of intermediate-acting insulin will cover the twenty-four-hour needs of the person who has diabetes. One dose of this type of insulin should be acceptable only for the person who needs a bedtime injection (NPH or lente insulin) in order to get the fasting glucose level within normal range. Only long-acting insulins that are peakless are chosen as basal insulins (e.g., Lantus). These basal insulins may be used with oral agents or short-acting or rapid-acting insulins before meals. For insulin-dependent people, the three-or-more-dose programs are being

Table 6.2 List of Insulins

ELI LILLY & CO.

Type	Name of Insulin	Source
Rapid-acting (Therapeutic action: onset 5–15 minutes, peak 30 minutes–1½ hours, duration 2–4 hours)	Humalog (lispro)	Designer
Short-acting (Therapeutic action: animal—onset 30 minutes–2 hours, peak 3–4 hours, duration 4–6 hours; human—onset 30 minutes–1 hour, peak 2–3 hours, duration 3–6 hours)	Iletin II R Humulin R	Pork (purified) Human
Intermediate-acting (Therapeutic action: animal—onset 4–6 hours, peak 8–14 hours, duration 26–30 hours; human—onset 2–4 hours, peak 4–10 hours, duration 10–16 hours)	Iletin II N Humulin N	Pork (purified) Human
(Therapeutic action: animal—onset 4–6 hours, peak 8–14 hours, duration 16–20 hours; human—onset 3–4 hours, peak 4–12 hours, duration 12–18 hours)	Iletin II L Humulin L	Pork (purified) Human
Long-acting (Therapeutic action: onset 6–10 hours, peak 16–18 hours, duration 18–20 hours)	Humulin U	Human
Mixture (Therapeutic action: onset ½–2 hours, peak 2–8 hours, duration 6–12 hours) (Humulin 70/30 is a mixture of 70 percent NPH and 30 percent regular; Humulin 50/50 is a mixture of 50 percent NPH and 50 percent regular)	Humulin 70/30 Humulin 50/50	Human Human
(Therapeutic action: onset 5–15 minutes/ 2 hours, peak 1 hour/4–10 hours, duration 3–4/10–16 hours)	72/25 (75 percent neutral protamine lispro/25 percent Humalog)	Designer

Table 6.2 List of Insulins, continued

NOVO-NORDISK

Type	Name of Insulin	Source
Short-acting (Therapeutic action: animal—onset 30 minutes–2 hours, peak 3–4 hours, duration 4–6 hours; human—onset 30 minutes–1 hour, peak 2–3 hours, duration 3–6 hours)	Regular Novolin R Velosolin	Pork (purified) Human Human (pump approved)
Intermediate-acting (Therapeutic action: onset 2–4 hours, peak 4–10 hours, duration 10–16 hours)	Novolin N	Human
(Therapeutic action: onset 4–6 hours, peak 8–14 hours, duration 16–20 hours)	Novolin L	Human
Rapid-acting (Therapeutic action: onset 5–15 minutes, peak 40–50 minutes, duration 2–3 hours)	Novolog (aspart)	Designer (pump approved)
Mixture (Therapeutic action: onset 15–30 minutes/2 hours, peak 2–8 hours, duration 2–4/12 hours; 70 percent Novalin N and 30 percent Novalin R)	Novolin 70/30 Novolin 70/30 mix	Human Designer

AVENTIS

Type	Name of Insulin	Source
Long-acting (Therapeutic action: 2–3 hours, peakless, duration 22½–26 hours) Glargine is a basal insulin that reaches the maximum of its ability in 2-3 hours and holds that level for approximately 22½ to 26 hours.	Lantus (glargine)	Designer

used more frequently. Twenty-four-hour control of the blood-glucose level is the goal. If less control is achieved, the possibility of reducing the risk of complications is lessened. The body normally produces a small amount of insulin continuously—basal insulin—and a burst of insulin with each intake of food (bolus). It is this pattern that needs to be duplicated with injectable insulin if control over the whole twenty-four-hour period is to be achieved.

Table 6.3 Therapeutic Goals for Blood Sugars

Premeal:	60–120 mg/dl (3.3–6.6 mmol)
2 hours after a meal:	less than 150 mg/dl (8 mmol)

For the pregnant woman (and ideally for others as they can tolerate it):

Premeal:	70–100 mg/dl (3.8–5.5 mmol)
2 hours after a meal:	less than 120 mg/dl (6.6 mmol), or less than 130 mg/dl (7.2 mmol)

(Average blood sugars should be 90–100 mg/dl [5–5.5 mmol].)

Rapid-Acting Insulin

Humalog (lispro) and Novolog (aspart) are presently the two rapid-acting insulins. These insulins have been genetically engineered to be more rapidly absorbed and utilized. Whereas human regular insulin takes thirty minutes to one hour to be absorbed, doesn't peak for two to three hours, and lasts three to six hours, rapid-acting insulins are absorbed in five to fifteen minutes, peak in about one hour (the same time that first-stage insulin release occurs after eating in the nondiabetic), and are gone in two to four hours. Humalog and Novolog are excellent insulins for keeping after-meal blood sugars under control. They are convenient to take since either one can be given right before or after the meal, and they don't overlap with the next meal, thereby avoiding premeal hypoglycemia. There are a couple of caveats with these insulins, however, that you and your health professional must observe:

1. These insulins are gone in two to four hours, so some longer-acting insulin may be needed to provide a background of insulin (i.e., basal insulin) to "cover the gaps." This could be one or two shots a day of NPH or lente insulin, one dose or a split dose of ultralente, or a single or split dose of lantus insulin. Sometimes people have been known to mix regular insulin with the Humalog for the coverage needed.

2. Since these insulins are more rapid in action, they may be gone before the next meal. Thus a premeal blood-sugar reading may not measure the action of the Humalog or Novolog insulin but instead measure the effect of the backup insulin. As the package inserts say, with these insulins you must measure the blood sugar two hours after the meal to determine the action and then adjust the dose of Humalog or Novolog as needed.

With these caveats, these insulins can help you avoid low blood-sugar episodes and add convenience, more physiological control, and much more flexibility to your insulin program and lifestyle.

Short-Acting Insulin

The short-acting insulins are regular, Iletin II R, Novolin R, and Humulin R. These insulins start working within thirty minutes, with the strongest, or peak, action occurring in two to four hours. The pharmacokinetic duration of action is from six to eight hours or longer, while the therapeutic duration of action is between four and eight hours. (Note: Semilente insulin, considered a short-acting insulin, has not been available in the United States since February 1994.)

Intermediate-Acting Insulin

The intermediate-acting insulins are Iletin II N, Novolin N, Humulin N, Iletin II L, Novolin L, NPH, and Humulin L. The human insulins start working in two to four hours, with peak action in four to twelve hours. The pharmacokinetic duration of action is reported to be eighteen to twenty hours or longer (the shortest therapeutic action, or pharmacodynamic action, of these insulins is reported to be ten to sixteen hours). Note that the human NPH insulins have a therapeutic duration of action closer to ten to twelve hours, while the pork or lente insulins have a duration of action closer to fourteen to sixteen hours.

Long-Acting Insulin

Long-acting insulins, such Humulin U, are being used as basal insulins, that is, ultralente has a slight peak. The pharmacodynamics appear to be less than twenty-four hours, so often the ultralente is split, with half given in the morning and half given in the evening. This insulin takes a long time to act (about eight hours), peaks in about eighteen hours, and has a pharmacokinetic action of thirty-six hours or more.

The second insulin in this category is called glargine (Lantus). It is described as having a "flat curve," as it rises to the onset of action in about one-and-a-half to three hours and then stays at that level of action for twenty-two-and-a-half to twenty-four hours pharmacodynamically and twenty-four to twenty-six hours pharmacokinetically. It is ideal as a basal insulin in that it can be given once or twice a day, but it may not be mixed with any of the present available insulins (pH of 4, more acid insulin, versus pH of 7, all other insulins). It must be given in its own syringe.

Long-acting insulins are used for a basal insulin effect (a little insulin every so many minutes), with doses (called boluses) of short-acting insulin given prior to each meal or large snack. This is a very effective way for many individuals to manage their diabetes. This regimen is especially useful with lispro or aspart insulin, which is ultrafast-acting and can be given before or right after a meal instead of thirty minutes beforehand, to get the best use of the rapid-acting insulins.

Premixed Insulin

Premixed insulins are also useful in specific instances. Eli Lilly & Co. has a 70/30 human mixture (Humulin 70/30—70 percent NPH and 30 percent regular) and a 50/50 insulin, and Novo-Nordisk also has a 70/30 insulin (Novolin 70/30). Pen-filled cartridges and prefilled cartridges are available. Europe has other combinations of insulin in addition to 70/30 and 50/50. So far, the Food and Drug Administration (FDA) in the United States has approved only the 70/30, the 50/50, the 75/25, and the 70/30 mixtures.

Methods of Insulin Delivery

Insulin may be delivered in one of several ways: under the skin (subcutaneous), into the muscle (intramuscular), sprayed through the skin, or delivered into the vein (intravenous). The instrument used for delivery of insulin may be a syringe/pen, syringe autoinjector, jet injector, IV (intravenous) infusion, or insulin infusion pump. Subcutaneous insulin is given only by syringe, pen, autoinjector, or jet injector (sprays insulin through the skin). When insulin is administered by vein, into the muscle, or with an infusion pump, only the short-acting (regular or crystalline) or rapid-acting insulins are given. (Only Velosolin and Novolog are approved by the FDA for use in pumps.) The fastest way to get insulin circulating through your body is to inject it into the vein. The

Table 6.4 Steps in Insulin Injection

1. Wash hands.
2. Clean bottle top.
3. Pull air into syringe equal to the amount of insulin to be given.
4. Push air into bottle from syringe.
5. Pull insulin into syringe (bubble free).
6. Clean skin.
7. Inject needle at 45° to 90° angle; short needles at 90°.
8. Pull out needle.
9. Apply mild pressure on site.

next fastest way is to have it delivered into the muscle. The peak action of intramuscular short-acting insulin is about one-and-a-half hours, rather than the two to four hours for insulin injected under the skin.

The important points about giving insulin subcutaneously are to ensure the cleanliness of the process and to give the correct amount at the right time (see Table 6.4). All parts of the procedure are important. However, while omitting certain steps will not have a detrimental effect on the blood-glucose levels, omitting other steps will. When getting insulin out of the bottle, first clean the top of the bottle, then replace the vacuum in which the insulin is manufactured by injecting into the bottle an amount of air that is equal to the amount of insulin to be removed. To be sure the correct amount of insulin is injected, you can do the following: check that the amount of air to be injected into the bottle is equal to the amount of insulin to be removed, check the amount of insulin in the syringe in relation to the dosage to be given, and check the syringe against the bottle to make sure that you have pulled the insulin from that specific bottle into the syringe. To ensure that the right bottle is chosen at the right time, color code the labels (for example, red for morning, orange for noon, green for suppertime, and blue for bedtime).

Mixing Insulins for Injection

If insulin is to be mixed in a syringe (see Table 6.5), the tops of both bottles are cleansed and air equal to the insulin to be removed is injected into each bottle. Once the air is placed into the short-acting insulin bottle (e.g., regular), the desired amount of insulin is withdrawn. The nee-

Table 6.5 Steps for Mixing Insulin in a Syringe

1. Wash hands.
2. Wipe off tops of both bottles.
3. Pull air into syringe equal to insulin desired.
4. Push air into bottles from syringe.
5. Pull insulin into syringe (bubble free) from bottle #1 (for example, Regular).
6. Pull insulin into syringe (bubble free) to total mark from bottle #2 (for example, NPH).
7. Clean skin.
8. Inject needle (45°–90° angle).
9. Pull out needle.
10. Apply mild pressure on site.

dle is then removed from that bottle and carefully placed into the other bottle. The insulin is very carefully withdrawn until the total amount of dosage is obtained in the syringe (for example, ten units of regular plus twenty units of NPH drawn up, in total, to the thirty-unit mark on the syringe).

This insulin should be administered within five minutes from the time it was initially mixed in the syringe or after a period of fifteen minutes after being mixed. Premixed insulin should not be kept in a syringe for longer than two weeks. Premixing of lente with regular insulin is not recommended unless it is administered immediately. Lente insulins cannot be premixed with NPH. Premixed NPH and regular (i.e., 70/30 and 50/50) are usable up to the date (shelf life) on the box. Humalog and Novolog should be mixed only with NPH, but some health professionals have suggested Humalog with regular (and immediately injecting it) to mimic the first stage (thirty minutes to one hour after eating) and second stage (two to three hours after eating) of insulin release in a nondiabetic person's response to food. Lantus may not be mixed with any nonacid insulins.

Insulin Injection Process

When it comes to giving a painless injection, the least amount of discomfort is experienced when the insulin is at room or body temperature and is given without any "drag" on the needle (that is, the needle either pierces tight skin or is rapidly pushed through the skin layer). Once the insulin has been administered at an even rate of speed, the needle should be quickly withdrawn at the same angle at which it was inserted. Applying mild pressure on the injection site for a minute or so will aid in keeping the insulin from leaking out onto the skin surface. (Some people use what is called Z-tracking: The needle is placed through the skin, the tip is moved to an angle, and the insulin is pushed in. On removal, the tip is moved back to its original location and is then pulled from the body. Such a technique is not usually necessary but can be helpful for those who experience a lot of "leaking.")

Insulin in use may be kept at room temperature for a month. However, damage to the insulin might occur if it is kept at a temperature greater than 80 degrees or below 40 degrees Fahrenheit. Due to temperature sensitivity, it is recommended that a bottle of Lantus (must be refrigerated) should not be used after twenty-eight days.

To prevent infection, the skin should be as clean as possible. To be sure of this, give the injection after a bath or shower, or wash the injection area with soap and water or with a cleansing wipe. The skin should be made tight by pinching a large fold of skin or, in the case of loose skin (such as might be found on the abdomen), pinching and pulling/stretching the skin so that the injection is given in the stretched area, not the pinched area.

The injection is given at an angle of 45 to 90 degrees, unless atrophy is to be treated, in which case a 20-degree angle is recommended. The angle depends on the thickness of the skin—the thicker the skin, the greater the angle. A younger child or elderly person would most likely need a 45-degree angle of injection, while a young or middle-aged adult would probably need a 90-degree angle. When short needles are used, there is a greater need to give a 90-degree injection.

Other Methods of Insulin Delivery

Abbott Laboratories' MediSense Product makes Precision Sure Dose syringes in 1 cc (100 units; ½-inch needle in 28 and 29 gauge), ½ cc (50 units), and ³⁄₁₀ cc (30 units) (the latter two available with ⅜-inch and ½-inch needles in 29 and 30 gauge). Aimsco makes Ultra Thin II, Maxi Comfort, and UniBody Ultra II syringes in 1 cc and ½ cc sizes with comparable needle lengths (except for the Ultra Thin II, which is available with a ⁵⁄₁₆-inch needle) and gauges as MediSense. Becton Dickinson manufactures Ultra-Fine II Short, Fine, and Fine IV syringes in 1 cc,

½ cc, and ³⁄₁₀ cc sizes. Their 1 cc syringe also includes a 30-gauge needle and is available in ½-inch and ⁵⁄₁₆-inch needle lengths. Can-Am Care
sells Monoject syringes. They come in Ultra Comfort Short and Ultra
Comfort 28- and 29-gauge needles. Needle length availability is ⅜-inch
and ⁵⁄₁₆-inch and the syringes are 1 cc, ½ cc, ³⁄₁₀ cc, and ¼ cc. Other syringes
are produced by Medicore (Lite Touch), UltiMed, Inc., UltiCare (Fine
and UltiCare Smooth), and Wal-Mart Pharmacies. While Medicore and
UltiCare have only ⁵⁄₁₆- or ½-inch needles on their syringes, Wal-Mart has
³⁄₁₀ cc syringes. Medicore does not produce a ³⁄₁₀ cc syringe at this time.

The short needles are for children and elderly people with thin skin
(i.e., 31 gauge; ³⁄₁₀-inch needle). Originally, they were not meant for
adults. All needles are now silicon coated to lubricate entry and prevent
discomfort.

Other Methods of Injection

Autoinjectors fit all sizes of insulin syringes. They include Becton Dickinson's Automatic Injector, Monoject's Injectomatic (distributed by Can-
Am Care), Autoject and Autoject 2 by Owens Mumford, Inc., Penmate
by Novo-Nordisk, Inject-Ease (Palco), and Instaject (Medicool, Inc.).
Autoject also holds the less available ³⁄₁₀ cc syringe. These injection
aids assist in getting the needle through the skin, with the person either
pushing the plunger in to administer the insulin or pressing a button
to shoot both the needle and the insulin into the skin. The costs vary
from $20 to $150.

The jet injectors are more expensive. They work by blowing the
insulin through the skin. Those presently available are the Activa-brand
products Advanta Jet and Advanta Jet ES (for tougher skin) and Gen-
tle Jet (designed for children). Equidyne Systems offers Injex 30, an injector that delivers from five to thirty units of insulin in a single or mixed
doses. Medi-Jector, produced by Medi-Ject Corporation, is reusable
for two to fifty units of all types of insulin. Vitajet 3, made by Bioject,
Inc., also delivers two to fifty units of various insulins. The depth of penetration may be regulated through adjustment of the nozzle on the jet
injector unit. Proper cleaning of the mechanism through which the insulin
is blown is a necessary step in the use of many of these instruments. Costs
range from about $500 to $900. Bottles or vials of insulin are used.

Medi-Ject and Vitajet are two needle-free systems that have started using disposable nozzles. The snap-and-click placement design "blows" the insulin through the skin. Learn more about these systems by visiting their websites at www.mediject.com or www.vitajet.com.

Insulin pens are another method of delivering insulin. Eli Lilly & Co. and Novo-Nordisk have made pens specific for their insulin in pre-filled or cartridge-filled forms, for example, Humalog Mix 75/25, Humalog, Humulin 70/30, and Humulin N; NovoPen 3 (one unit), NovoPen Jr (half unit), InNovo (doser and timer), InDuo (doser and monitor), Flexipen (forward and backward dial ability), and Innolet (large dial). Figure 6.1 shows examples of penfilled and prefilled insulin pens. All pens use screw-on needles. These pens are also available through Owen Mumford, Inc. (the Autopen), Disetronic Medical Systems, and Becton Dickinson. Becton Dickinson and Novo-Nordisk make ultrafine pens and short needles.

Pens may be ordered through your local pharmacy. Cartridges may include 150 to 300 units of insulin. These cartridges are disposable. Novo-Nordisk's and Eli Lilly's prefilled pens are also disposable. Cartridges and pens from Eli Lilly and Novo-Nordisk are very popular in Europe and are becoming increasingly popular in the United States as more people go to a multiple-dose regimen. They are especially useful

Figure 6.1 Prefilled Pen Devices

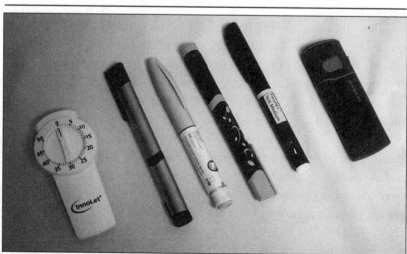

Figure 6.2 Historical Changes in Insulin-Infusion Systems

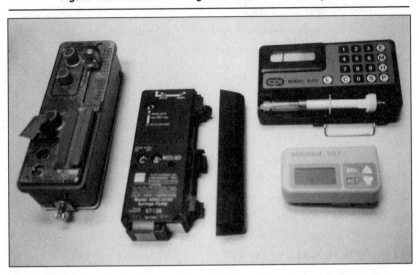

for doses of insulin needed when a person is away from home (i.e., at work, school, or a restaurant, or when traveling).

Insulflon (made by MEDgenesis) is an aid in multiple-injection therapy. The multiple daily injections are given through a diaphragm connected to a small plastic tube that has been placed beneath the skin with the use of a needle guide. This placement is usually done on a two-to-three-day to weekly basis.

Insulin pumps are also becoming more popular. Over time, these pumps have become smaller and more sophisticated (see Figure 6.2).

Many companies have made insulin pumps in the past. Today four companies market insulin pumps in the United States. These companies are MiniMed Technologies, Disetronic Medical Systems, Animas, and Deltec Cosmos. MiniMed currently markets the MiniMed 508 pump and the more advanced Paradigm (see Figure 6.3), an insulin pump. These pumps deliver multiple basals (forty-eight profiles), boluses, and a "square wave"—an increased amount of insulin given over a number of minutes to hours and useful for larger and/or longer meals. Disetronic currently markets the H-TRON Plus, the D-TRON, the D-TRON Plus (which communicates with the Dialog Pump Programming Tool), and the Dahedi. The H-TRON Plus delivers zero to ninety-nine units an hour with twenty-four profiles. Its "sister," the

Figure 6.3 MiniMed 508 Insulin Pump

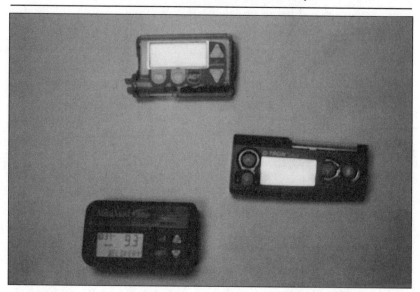

D-TRON, has a range ability to deliver zero to twenty-five units and also has twenty-four basal rates. The Dahedi is the smallest pump, delivering zero to six units an hour. It has twenty-four basal rates plus fourteen different alarms. The Animas 5-1000 and 1000A have twelve basal rates and the 1000 has a range of 0.1 to 4.9 units per hour to the 1000A's 0.1 to 9.9 units per hour. The Animas IR1000 is even more user-friendly than past models with carb counting and insulin choices. It has a "toggle and click" memory. The Deltec Cosmo has carbohydrate calculations and suggested insulin corrections.

All pumps manufactured now have either a 1.0 unit or a 0.5 unit as the smallest bolus capable of delivery. All pumps are also now waterproof within defined expectations. These highly technical instruments administer a basal insulin (insulin at certain small intervals throughout a twenty-four-hour period), plus an automatic or manual dose before each meal or at other desired times.

Individuals using these instruments must be knowledgeable, stable, and motivated. For safety's sake, blood-glucose tests must be taken four to six times or more each day. Having consistently more normal blood-glucose levels means that fewer physical signals might be felt if the blood-sugar levels drop to hypoglycemic levels. Such tight control

also may lead to the possibility that the body will not take the opportunity to attain and maintain adequate amounts of stored glucose for
emergency use. But the more normal the blood-glucose levels, the less
risk of developing eye, nerve, kidney, and some heart complications.

Plugging of the tubing, lack of battery power, running out of insulin,
and abscess formation under the skin are some of the potential problems of pumps. Presently, Velosolin, Humalog, and Novolog insulins
are used for pumps. The use of purified and designer insulins has
decreased the plugging problem. An alarm now sounds if the battery
power is getting low. There is also an alarm if the insulin volume is low
or if the insulin volume has stopped. Skin infection and abscesses are
much less common now than in the early years of pump therapy due to
better insertion techniques, better skin cleansers, and plastic needles.
Care must still be observed and the site changed at frequent intervals
(every two to three days is recommended). Overall, pumps have become
safer and more user-friendly.

A continuous monitoring system (CMS) is a glucose sensor that may
be worn for three days in order to determine if the blood sugars are at
the optimum level between boluses and on certain basals. (Frequently
checking blood-glucose levels is necessary to offset the drift of the
machine.) Averaging out this information can lead to more suitable basal
and bolus decisions.

The GlucoWatch monitors blood sugar over a twelve-hour period.
Blood-glucose readings may be obtained every ten minutes after the initial setup time of 1½ hours and one finger stick (blood sugar test).

Special Instruments for Insulin Administration

Equipment is available to assist the partially sighted or blind individual
in reading the syringe. Insul-eze from Palco Labs, Magni-Guide from
Becton Dickinson, Tru-Hand from Whittier Medical, Hypoviewer from
HypOview, and the clip-on Syringe Magnified from Apothecard Products are some of the items available. A needle guide called Holdease is
available through Meditec, Inc. Voice synthesizers are available through
Roche (Accu-Chek Voicemate), Science Products (Digi-Voice Deluxe
and Touch-n-Talk Profile for the One Touch I, Profile, Basic, and Sure-
Step meters), and Myna Corporation (Voice Touch, which also works
with the One Touch II or One Touch Profile).

Count-a-dose (Jordan Medical), Insulgage (Meditec), and Insul-Cap and Load-Matic (Palco Labs) provide assistance by making it easier to accurately load the syringe and deliver the insulin. The Novolin pen has clickers to help in calculating the insulin dose, while Innolet has an "egg timer" capability and a low cost. Many of these products may be purchased through the American Foundation for the Blind or directly from the manufacturer.

There are other insulin-delivery machines currently being tested. There will be a need for more advances in insulins and oral medications, along with delivery devices, until there is a cure for this potentially devastating syndrome of diseases.

7

What Is Important
About Exercise?

Exercise has great importance as part of the medical management of the person who has diabetes mellitus. The best exercise program is one in which aerobic activity is done for a period of twenty to thirty minutes on a daily or every-other-day basis.

Benefits of Exercise

There are many benefits of exercise, and they far outweigh the risks. Some of these benefits are improved heart and breathing actions. Another common benefit is the increase in muscular strength and endurance. There is a buildup of lean body mass and a decrease in body fat. The range of motion and the flexibility of the arms and legs are improved. Triglycerides and cholesterol are lowered. High-density lipoproteins (HDLs—the "good guys") are increased, while low-density lipoproteins (LDLs—the "bad guys") are decreased. Blood-pressure control is improved. Depression is decreased. The pain threshold is increased. Both self-image and self-esteem are improved, and, most important, a sense of well-being is achieved and enhanced.

There are benefits that are even more specific to diabetes management. Some of these are the increased sensitivity of the cell-receptor site to insulin. This sensitivity is noted as a decline in blood-glucose levels due to the improved use of insulin by the cells. The result is a reduction in the total insulin needed.

As exercise is maintained, there is a prolonged blood-glucose-lowering effect. Extensive short-term exercise may even result in lowered blood-glucose levels over a period of twenty-four to thirty-six hours. The Diabetes Type 2 Prevention Trial found exercise has an effect on the length of beta-cell function. These factors lead, directly and indirectly, to a decreased risk for atherosclerosis (a type of blood vessel/heart disease).

Aerobic exercise can be low, moderate, or high in intensity. It may be rhythmic, but it must be continuous—that is, while walking at varying rates is fine, walking, then stopping, then walking is not aerobic. Exercise must be of a certain duration (a minimum of thirty minutes three times a week, or twenty minutes five to six times a week). The major fuels used for aerobic exercise are glucose and free fatty acids. Good aerobic exercises are swimming, walking, rowing, cycling, and dancing (see Appendixes F and G for information on calorie burning). Cross-country (Nordic) skiing is the most effective of all aerobic exercises. Notice that jogging and other high-impact or "severe" aerobics have not been placed on this list. There have been too many risks found with such exercise; for the diabetic in particular, the risks outweigh the benefits. Therefore, walking or other low-impact aerobic exercise is recommended.

For an exercise to be aerobic, the heart rate must be at least 50 percent above the resting heart rate. The ceiling level is 75 to 80 percent. The ideal range is between 50 and 75 percent. (Various books give different figures. The common target range recommended is from 60 to 80 percent.)

To determine your target zone or ideal range, first subtract your age from 220. Then multiply this number by 60 percent (or another number, depending on a recommendation by your health care professional) to obtain your threshold level (the lower number of the range of beats per minute that you should aim for during your exercise period). Multiplying the same number by 80 percent will give you your ceiling level. You should aim to maintain your heart rate in this "ideal" range for twenty to thirty minutes (see Figure 7.1). (To feel your heartbeat, place your second and third fingers on the inner side of your wrist or on your neck about three inches below the bottom of your ear.)

Figure 7.1 Target Zone

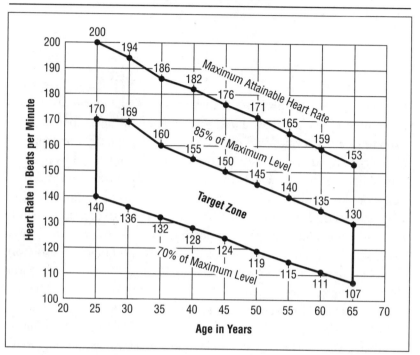

Since you are unable to determine your heart rate every minute unless you have a monitor in place, you can gain a rough estimate of how hard you are exercising by using the "Borg Scale of Perceived Exertion." The scale goes from six to twenty. Less than six means sleep or a resting state, while twenty means activity to the point of fatigue. Seven is very, very light activity, nine is light, and eleven is somewhat light. Nineteen is very, very hard, seventeen is very hard, fifteen is hard, and thirteen is somewhat hard. You would try to exercise in the range of twelve to sixteen, or the aerobic-intensity level.

Activities such as weight lifting, gymnastics, and some other sports-related activities (e.g., wrestling) are isokinetic exercises. This type of exercise uses glycogen or stored glucose as the major source of fuel. Activities of this type are intermittent, of short duration, and usually quite intense. They are called anaerobic (the person doesn't increase oxygen intake much over usual levels, unlike in aerobic exercise). Anaerobic activities do not offer as much benefit to the person who has diabetes, and in fact they may raise the blood pressure to the point of putting the body at risk.

Precautions in Exercising

Starting any exercise program requires taking some precautions, especially if you have diabetes. First, you must be in the proper shape to exercise. Have your health professional evaluate your present condition and recommend any necessary exercise restrictions (such as times or physical states during which you should not exercise). Unless certain heart or eye conditions exist, it is likely that no restrictions will be recommended. With blood-glucose testing, you can determine before exercising whether your blood-glucose level is too high or too low to exercise. If your blood-glucose level is less than 60 mg/dl (3.3 mmol), do not exercise. If the level is greater than 250 mg/dl (13.8 mmol), check the urine for ketones; if ketones are present, do not exercise. The reason for this is that exercise is a stressor to the body. If the body is "sick"—represented by blood-glucose levels of 250 mg/dl (13.8 mmol) or greater and by the presence of ketones—exercise would only make the body "sicker" (see Figure 7.2), as might a blood sugar of 300 mg/dl (16.6 mmol) or more without ketones.

Calories need to be adjusted to take exercise into account. The best time to exercise is approximately twenty minutes to one hour after a meal. This allows the food to settle before exercising and gives you the advantage of having some readily available glucose. If the exercise is to be of low intensity or short duration and the blood sugar is above 100 mg/dl (5 to 5.5 mmol), then no extra snack is needed. If the exercise is carried out over a thirty-minute period or longer, then a snack is usually advised (this is more appropriate for high-intensity exercise). For high-intensity exercise, a snack would be eaten beforehand, with another snack eaten every thirty to sixty minutes. Some form of fast-acting simple sugar and an added snack food should be carried at all times. It can be eaten to treat an insulin reaction or to give yourself an energy boost or raise your blood-glucose level after completing the exercise period.

If you have Type 2 diabetes, and especially if you are also overweight, you do not need to eat extra calories for exercising unless

Figure 7.2 Warning Signs That May Accompany Exercise

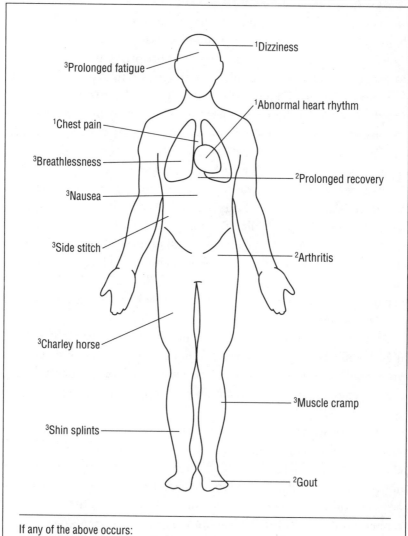

If any of the above occurs:

[1] Discontinue the exercise program.
[2] Try a suggested remedy briefly (such as warmth to the site or mild gradual stretching to relieve a muscle cramp). If unsuccessful, contact your physician.
[3] You can probably handle it yourself.

your blood-glucose level drops below normal (the usual between-meal snacks should be continued).

People with Type 1 diabetes may choose to lower insulin levels before the exercise period rather than increase food intake when they exercise heavily. This would be most appropriate if you desired to lose weight. For a growing child, a teenager, or an active adult, more food (to the level of amounts tolerated) might be the better choice. Some people may not be physically able to eat the number of increased calories needed. Therefore, they might increase calories as well as decrease insulin prior to the time of activity. Such determinations should be made on a one-to-one basis with your health professional.

Before exercising, note the time you last ate or last had an injection. If you are relating the time of exercise to the last injection, then you need to consider the type of insulin, the dosage, the peak and duration of its action, and the site of the injection. Insulin injected into an arm or leg that is used actively during the exercise is bound to be absorbed more rapidly. You would not want to exercise at the peak action time of an insulin without taking special precautions. Note what type of exercise you will be doing and how long you will be doing it.

Be sure that you do not hold your breath during your exercise activities. If you have any eye damage, do not get into a position that places your head lower than your heart. Also with eye damage, don't do any type of exercise that puts strain on your upper body, such as lifting weights.

Exercise with a partner. Teach this person how to treat an insulin reaction so that you have backup protection. Be aware of whether the exercise you are doing is part of your regular routine or if it is over and above what you usually do. Notice whether you are having any pains, aches, or other discomfort. Before you sit down, check that your pulse rate is less than 100 beats per minute. Recheck your pulse rate to be sure it is not going above the ceiling level. Be sure you do not exercise when it is too hot or too cold; overheating or becoming chilled can make anyone ill. Wear appropriate clothing (loose cotton clothing, with two pairs of socks and good-fitting shoes).

Any symptoms of insulin reaction mean that you need to stop exercising immediately and treat the insulin reaction. If you do not have extreme symptoms, for example, very weak and shaky, with double vision, check your blood-glucose levels so that you will learn how much exercise, and at what intensity, leads to such a response. Any severe insulin reaction means that you should do no more exercise that day, since the body needs time to recover.

Check your blood sugar about thirty minutes after exercising to be sure that you are not developing hypoglycemia. Eat a small snack if your blood glucose is below 80 mg/dl (4.4 mmol) after exercising.

Stretching before and after exercising reduces muscle tightness. You must be relaxed when you stretch; if you are not, you can do more harm than good. You should stretch slowly and in a sustained manner. The recommended time for the stretching of each of the arms and legs is ten to thirty seconds. As you stretch, your breathing should be slow, even, and rhythmic. The major precaution to take is to be sure not to bounce on a stretch, but instead to sustain the stretch for the recommended number of seconds. Be sure that you stretch each part of the body equally.

One more caveat: If your eyes have been treated by laser, you need to be careful in the choice of exercises you do for physical fitness. Exercise should not be done in a position that places the eyes below the level of the heart. If the head is placed lower than the heart in an exercise, there will be an increase in blood pressure. An example of such an exercise would be touching your toes.

The "Exercise Prescription"

The exercise prescription involves four factors:

1. The activity you choose
2. The frequency with which you participate in it
3. The intensity of your participation
4. The duration of the activity

These choices are based on your physical fitness, as determined by the assessment of your physical state. For the frequency, determine whether you are going to exercise three, four, or more times a week. Aim for a minimum of four times per week. Do not allow more than two days in a row to pass without taking some opportunity to exercise. Start slowly—every other day is recommended. Then add more days as tolerated.

The intensity is determined by your target heart rate (the pulse rate above the threshold and below the ceiling). If you are able to sing or talk while you are exercising, then you can assume you are exercising at the proper intensity. Remember the Borg Scale of Perceived Exertion? What is the range of your perceived exertion scale?

The older you are, the more slowly you should start the activity. Even starting with as short a time as three minutes (or, for the very elderly, just one minute) is wise. Gradually increase the time until you reach a goal of twenty to thirty minutes. If your goal is to reduce body fat, you must exercise for forty-five minutes or longer. Determine what you can tolerate, then add anywhere from one to five minutes each week until you have reached your goal.

Since there are many types of activities to choose from, you don't need to do the same type of exercise every day. Whatever exercise you choose for a given day, be sure it is done continuously and rhythmically (that is, at the same rate or at varying speeds but without completely stopping), that it involves large muscle groups, and that it is enjoyable! If you are bored with the exercise, do some other type of exercise. Boredom may become an obstacle leading to inactivity. On the other hand, don't overload yourself with activities to the point that you become burned out.

Focus on your goals of cardiovascular endurance, muscular strength, flexibility, and improved diabetes control—and be sure to have fun in the process.

8

What About Hygiene?

Daily care is one way to prevent sources of infection that lead to the increase of blood-glucose levels in the body. Daily care involves a number of practices. This chapter will focus on the practices of daily hygiene. These practices involve dental care, skin care, foot care, eye care, and care related to sexually related activities.

Dental Care

Numerous people have reported that once they had healed from having an abscessed tooth, their gingivitis (gum disease) had been cured, or they had a large cavity filled, their blood sugar became more normal. Any source of infection will "push" the blood sugar up. Therefore, keeping the teeth clean, massaging the gums, fighting plaque, and seeing your dentist every six months or as directed will directly or indirectly aid in controlling your blood-glucose levels.

First, you need to know what is recommended for good dental care (see Table 8.1). People with diabetes, especially older people, should see their dentist more frequently than every six months. If a person has dentures, observations should be made for any inflammation of the gums, with any such inflammation reported to the dentist. Teeth should be brushed, or at least the mouth should be rinsed, after every meal or snack. The major times to brush your teeth are on awakening and before going to sleep. Before going to bed, flossing is a must. Brushing reaches only

Table 8.1 Steps in Dental Care

1. Brush teeth at least twice a day with a circular, scrubbing motion.
2. Floss at least once a day, making sure the floss reaches the gum line between the teeth.
3. If plaque is a problem for you, use a plaque-loosening solution before brushing.
4. See your dentist every six months or as directed.

three sides of the tooth, but the tooth has five sides. Flossing reaches those other two sides. Gum massage is also helpful. This can be done with a water pick or with a rubber tip. Placing this tip under the gum line stimulates the flow of circulating blood and assists in ridding the mouth of debris that might have worked beneath the gum line. Flossing usually catches this, but sometimes it doesn't. (Note: To be most helpful, flossing must include the base of the tooth and the area under the gum line.)

If you have a problem with plaque, prerinsing with a plaque-loosening solution is recommended. Many toothpastes also contain ingredients to fight plaque, tartar, or both. The mechanical action of the toothbrush is your best ally in fighting plaque and massaging the gums. The old "from the top of the tooth down" technique has been replaced with the circular or round movement of the brush at the gum line and over the tooth surface.

If any dental surgery is to be performed, blood-glucose levels should be as normal as possible beforehand. The outcome will be better, that is, healing will occur at a more normal rate. Antibiotics may be started a few days before the surgical procedure to better support the prevention of infection.

The "quiet occurrence" of gingivitis should also be noted. If you notice any bleeding when you brush your teeth (and you are brushing at least twice a day), suspect gingivitis. Severe gingivitis can lead to loosening or loss of teeth and, if it goes under the gum line, bone involvement. Proper dental care and good nutrition, along with normal blood-glucose levels, are the best methods of preventing gingivitis.

Skin Care

Skin care is most associated with the simple act of bathing. Surprisingly, there can be both too much and too little use of water. Soaking the body can lead to tissue breakdown, while lack of cleanliness can lead to local infections. Drink plenty of water unless told to do otherwise.

Poor blood-glucose control may increase or reveal such conditions as necrobiosis lipoidica diabeticorum, a skin condition that looks much like scar tissue. Individuals with this problem often note that the scarred areas look more "angry" when their blood-glucose levels are higher. Other skin conditions associated with diabetes are also easier to notice with higher blood sugars. For example, xanthoma—a skin condition in which what looks like yellow pimples appear on the skin—may appear. When these pimples are seen, elevated lipid levels (fat levels) are found in the blood. Lowering the blood-glucose levels also results in a noticeable lowering of the lipid levels.

If there are frequent boils, carbuncles, or localized infections, high blood sugar and poor skin care should be noted. The sites should be cultured so that the appropriate medication may be given. Until the infections are under control, it is possible that there will be a greater need for insulin.

The need for more insulin may also be true for a yeast infection called candidiasis. Candidiasis may be found in the mouth, under the arms, under fatty folds of the skin, and in genital areas. Local and general medication (medication taken by mouth) may be prescribed. This infection occurs less frequently with lowered blood-glucose levels. If blood-glucose levels are not monitored, the person should suspect high blood-glucose levels the majority of the time if such conditions are noted.

When the blood-glucose levels are controlled, there is less chance that such skin and mouth conditions will occur. If diabetes control is accompanied with good skin hygiene, with bathing done on a daily or every-other-day basis, skin infections should be minimal or nonexistent. (Note: Older people in particular may have difficulty with dry skin conditions if bathing is frequent during the drier winter months.)

Foot Care

Using powders when the skin is moist and lotions when it is dry are the general instructions for skin care, and they are particularly important when it comes to the feet. Good care of the feet is necessary to prevent the breaking down of skin areas, since such areas could become sites for infection (see Table 8.2).

The feet are a very vulnerable part of the body when it comes to injury or infection. Walking barefoot and having a lack of feeling set the feet up for some serious problems. If circulation to the feet is poor, the blood flow is not adequate to meet the needs of the healing process. Poor circulation also leads to a lack of healthy nerves. Less-than-adequate circulation may be due directly or indirectly to high blood-glucose levels, which can affect the major blood vessels or the cells that act as "insulation" around the nerves. When this insulation is no longer present, the nerves short-circuit (just like two uninsulated wires), and the result is pain, numbness, or both.

Care of the feet is easier for some than for others. An overweight person may have difficulty seeing the bottoms of his or her feet. Careful and daily assessment of the feet is one of the major ways to prevent problems and to ensure that any problems noted are reported early. You should observe your feet for signs of infection (reddened or swollen areas, pus, a red streak up the leg, or pain [if the nerves are functioning adequately]); for corns and, especially, calluses (which can hide tissue breakdown, as this may start under the surface of the callus); for nails that are too long and need trimming; and for areas experiencing pressure (which may indicate that your shoes are ill fitting). Toenails may be sites for fungal infections. Yellowed nails may be treated by medication taken internally (Sporonex, Diflucan) or applied externally (Penlac). When people need help in inspecting their feet, a flexible or bendable neck mirror may be purchased.

Table 8.2 Steps in Foot Care

1. Inspect feet daily.
2. Wash feet daily.
3. Dry between toes.
4. Use powder (when damp) and lotion (when dry) and rub in place.
5. Wear clean socks daily.
6. Keep feet warm by wearing warm socks.
7. Cut toenails as directed.
8. Use a buffing pad on calluses after bathing.
9. See a podiatrist for stubborn corns and calluses.
10. Have your physician or other health professional examine your feet four times per year to check the pulse, temperature, and color in order to determine whether your circulation is adequate. You will also be tested for reflexes, vibratory sense, and responses to sharp and dull objects (or just the ability to feel an object touch the foot) at least once a year.

Besides the sole, an area of the foot that is often missed is the area between the toes. This warm, moist place may harbor infection or breakdown of tissue. Athlete's foot is also most commonly found here.

Cleanliness of the feet is the next thing to emphasize. If the feet are injured, it stands to reason that the possibility of infection will be less if they are clean.

Seeing a podiatrist (foot doctor) for foot problems such as calluses or corns is next in the sequence of care. Calluses that have become enlarged should be filed by a podiatrist. Corn development should be prevented, but if corns do occur you should see a podiatrist. (Note: Ill-fitting shoes may be the problem; daily changes of shoes and checking for pressure areas from the shoes worn are helpful.) "Young" calluses or corns can be rubbed, loosened, or removed after a bath.

Toenail-cutting guidelines are as follows: The toenail should be cut following the line of the toe. This is usually stated as "cut the nails straight across," but in line with the top of the toe. File the sharp corners until smooth. The curving of the cut into the edges of the toe is not recommended unless the person has problems with ingrown toenails. Ingrown toenails can best be treated by a podiatrist.

Other things to consider are the shoes you choose to wear. Shoes should be made of leather (so they will breathe), and they should fit well. They should be broken in slowly (that is, worn for a few hours the first day, a few more the next day, and so on, until there are no noticeable pressure areas and no discomfort). As noted before, shoes should be changed every day or every other day, whenever possible. Socks should be clean and fit the foot properly. Any creases or wrinkles may prove to be a pressure site after the shoe is in place. Feet should be kept warm with warm socks rather than with a heating pad or a hot-water bottle.

If you are bedridden, exercises for the feet will be helpful in maintaining good circulation to the feet. These exercises should involve elevating and lowering the feet, and activity of the feet involving circular and up-and-down movements (called Buerger exercises). Walking is also good exercise for the feet, but only if the shoes worn fit well and have good support around the ankles and arches. Walking barefoot is not considered a good thing to do (whether the person has diabetes or not), since there is just too much of a chance that the feet will be injured.

Some people do not consider checking the insides of their shoes for any foreign objects before putting them on. However, sensation may be lost in the foot, and repeated pressure or other injury of the foot—such as that caused by a tack stuck in the bottom of the shoe, or a small toy or other object in the shoe—may lead to problems without the person's really knowing this has happened.

If an injury, such as a cut or scratch, should occur, any alcohol-based product will just burn the tissues and impede (or slow) the healing process. Soap and water works best, followed by careful drying (especially between the toes).

To review: Feet should be washed daily. The water in which they are washed should be warm, not hot. The feet should be dried completely. If the skin is dry, lotion should be applied; if sweaty, powder should be used (be sure the powder or lotion is rubbed in well if used between the toes). After the daily washing, while the skin is still softened, callused areas should be buffed to aid in removing the dead skin, and toenails should be cut as directed. If feet need to be warmed, this can be accomplished by putting on warm socks. Going barefoot is discouraged. Feet should be inspected daily. If problems are noted (for example, infections or pressure areas), you should contact a podiatrist or other health professional.

There is a saying that if you treat your feet right, they will treat you right. This is especially true when you have diabetes.

Eye Care

Eye care is also a part of hygiene. Many illnesses, such as colds and flu, are passed on by contact of the hands with either the mouth or the eyes. You should wash your hands before you do anything related to the eyes. If you wear contact lenses, be sure to wash your hands before handling the lenses to prevent eye infections. Any eye infection should be treated promptly. Pink eye (an acute, highly contagious type of conjunctivitis—inflammation of the white parts of the eye) can result in blindness if not treated correctly.

For the person who does not have diabetes, routine eye exams should be done every two years. For the person with diabetes, the eyes should be checked every year or even more frequently, as recommended by the ophthalmologist or retinologist. Note: Because optometrists used to be trained primarily to fit glasses, in the past people with diabetes mellitus were advised to see an ophthalmologist or retinologist instead. The reasoning for this guidance was the potential for eye disease with elevated blood-glucose levels. However, optometrists are now educated to look for eye diseases and even to take retinal photographs to look for diabetes-related eye diseases. If a disease is found, the optometrist will refer you to an ophthalmologist or retinologist for treatment.

It is recommended that anyone given a diagnosis of Type 2 diabetes have an eye exam immediately, with retinal photographs taken. The person who is newly diagnosed with Type 1 diabetes should have retinal photographs taken after five years of diagnosis. However, it would be wise to have such an eye evaluation four to six weeks after blood-glucose levels were controlled to determine a baseline to be used for later comparison or for any change in glasses.

Eye exercises are another consideration for good eye care. While this area is somewhat controversial, many people feel that exercises that involve the eye muscles can strengthen the eyes. For example, when you are doing close work, every fifteen to twenty minutes look into the distance and alternate with looking close ten times.

Eyes are a very precious part of the body. Your vision can be stable and can last a lifetime if your eyes are well cared for. If treatment is needed, it should be administered as early as possible.

Sexually Related Hygiene

Human sexuality involves the sensual feelings, the reproductive process, gender identification, general cleanliness, prevention of infections in the genital area, and sexual behavior. The genital area can be a source of infection, which can cause blood-glucose elevation. Also, if a person does not feel that he or she is functioning well enough sexually, blood-glucose elevation can occur. Pregnancy (which will be discussed in Chapter 10 under the heading of "Intermediate Complications") is also a cause of higher blood-glucose levels. Finally, confusion in gender identification may result in stress, which is associated with elevation of blood-glucose levels.

A person's mental health can be affected if he or she becomes worried about diabetes-related problems of decreased sexual functioning. Rest assured that this dysfunction or inability to have an erection or orgasm is probably more mental than physical. If you read some information and suspect you may be having such dysfunction, you are likely to focus on performance rather than enjoyment; this focus will then affect your functioning. If you find that your focus is on your performance, get some assistance from a therapist accredited by the American Association of Sex Educators, Counselors, and Therapists. If you still have some questions, speak with your health professional. There are specific tests that can aid in determining whether your sexually associated problems are psychological or physical in origin. Most of the time, you will find that no physical problem exists.

Where physical problems do exist, much can now be done with prostheses (silastic implants that are permanently rigid, semirigid, or inflatable), with assistive devices (such as a vacuum pump and a Velcro belt to place at the base of the erect penis or the use of injections), or with hormone (testosterone) or chemical therapy. Women who have loss of libido can be treated with low doses of the male hormone testosterone, which stimulates libido. Men with low testosterone levels can also be treated with it. Women with dryness of the vagina can use a variety of lubricants, one of which is Albolene, a water soluble, greaseless, nonirritating lubricant (labeled as a cosmetic cleanser). MUSE (medicated urethral system erection) is a chemical, called a *prostaglandin*, to be placed as a small suppository in the urethra with the use of a plastic applicator. It works by dilating the arteries and the smooth muscle in the penis. Return blood flow is slowed and/or stopped, and an erection occurs. Couples using this therapy have at least a 65 percent response over those receiving a fake (placebo) suppository.

The newest drug therapy development is Viagra. This drug is a blood vessel dilator that dilates the blood vessels all over the body, thus producing such side effects as headache and dizziness. Persons prone to heart attacks or those who are taking other blood vessel dilators such as nitroglycerin, should not use this drug, as too much dilation can lead to a heart attack. Viagra is taken as a pill, by mouth, in doses of 50 to 150 mg about one hour before sex to produce an erection that can last as long as three to four hours. Viagra is currently being tested on women, as it may cause clitoral erection and thus increase sensitivity and orgasmic potential. Anecdotal experience suggests that it works in women, but scientific data are not yet available, although studies are under way.

If a problem is suspected and you feel uncomfortable in bringing up the subject of sexual discomfort (some women may feel discomfort with intercourse from having a dry vaginal area due to hyperglycemia or to aging) or performance, write it down and present the problem to your health professional in written form. If you discuss such problems, you will find that the information will be handled confidentially, as any other body function would be discussed. If other health professionals or students are in the room, ask to speak to your health professional privately. Describe what you think is happening. Your health professional knows what questions to ask to assist you in finding the best solution to the problem, if one is found to exist.

For any treatment, the health professional will take into account your own beliefs and attitudes and your physical developmental history. He or she can assist you in making changes or offer an appropriate referral.

Your participation in all hygiene measures and your early reporting of any infection or injury will help your health care team to keep you in the best possible physical condition. The result will be that you will feel better about yourself and about your health.

9

How Is Diabetes Monitored?

Diabetes is known to cause high blood-glucose levels, but how do you know to what extent this has occurred to you? When insulin is too low and glucose levels are too high, glucose is not getting into the cells. How do you know to what extent glucose has not entered the cells and, therefore, to what extent you need another source of energy (fatty acids in a form called *ketone bodies*)? Testing for blood-glucose levels and for ketones in the urine is the short-term answer. For the longer-term answer, testing is done for fructosamine or glycosylated serum protein (such tests show control over the past two or more weeks) and glycosylated hemoglobin. A glycosylated hemoglobin test, especially hemoglobin A1c, the most common test prescribed, shows control over a period of two to three months by indicating the percent of glucose attached to the protein in the red blood cell (life span of 120 days) that is above normal.

Without such testing, people with diabetes cannot know whether their diabetes is really controlled. Regular testing allows you to know the ongoing status of the disease, but just at the times of testing. Keeping blood-sugar (glucose) levels as normal as possible is the best way to reduce the risk by potentially preventing or delaying vascular (blood-vessel) or neurological (nerve) complications. High blood-sugar (glucose) levels lead to damage of the body cells. It is known that if animals have a blood-sugar level of 150 mg/dl (8.3 mmol) or more, they develop blood-vessel, kidney, nerve, and eye diseases. It is also known that Pima

Indians with diabetes who participated in one study, and who maintained a blood-sugar (glucose) level of 165 mg/dl (9.2 mmol) or higher, developed these same complications of the disease. The conclusion reached by these and many other studies is that the higher the blood sugar is allowed to be, the greater the possibility of physical problems. Unless blood-sugar levels are controlled most of the time, partial efforts are apparently of little value.

Frequency of Testing

Studies in various parts of the country have indicated that a single blood-glucose measurement, done in the physician's office every few weeks or months, is still the most common method of diabetes management in the United States. However, other studies have demonstrated the futility of this type of management, and more and more people are being treated by physicians who weigh the results of self-monitoring of blood glucose (SMBG) and glycosylated hemoglobin of some form (such as HgA1c, which is less influenced by immediate high and low blood sugar excursions, or HgA1, which measures A1a, A1b, and A1c), rather than having a single blood-glucose measurement done.

The philosophy of obtaining a fasting or postmeal blood-glucose measurement at a clinic visit is that blood-glucose levels are relatively stable and that the measurement obtained thus reflects the level over the past few weeks and predicts the level for the next few weeks. *Nothing could be further from the truth.* We reviewed a patient's chart recently and found the following office blood sugars at three-month intervals, looking only at fasting blood sugars, of 217, 67, 197, 46, and 125 mg/dl. If management was based on these measurements, the medicine would have been increased at blood sugars of 217 and 197, decreased at 67 and 46, and kept the same at 125. In actual fact, in comparison with the HgA1c (6.8 percent), the blood-sugar (glucose) overall averages (fasting and two hours after each meal) obtained through self-testing were about the same for each visit (averaging less than 150 mg/dl, or 8.3 mmol), indicating that there was only a need to change the diabetes medication at specific times of the day. Blood sugar is constantly changing, so a blood-sugar test in a clinic's office measures the blood sugar only for that moment in time.

Table 9.1 Instructions for Testing Blood Sugar

1. Wash hands.
2. Place strip into the machine and watch indicator for placing blood to strip.
3. Pierce finger and obtain a drop of blood. The type of drop of blood is dependent on the type of strip you are using (i.e., "hanging drop" versus small drop for strips that draw blood into the strip—capillary action).
4. Place blood on or at the side of the strip.
5. Read results at end of test time and respond as needed.
6. Record results or refer to results in the memory of your meter at least one to two times a week.

The frequency of self–blood testing suggests that testing is different for different clinics. Researchers have shown that the more testing done (and responded to), the better the control and the fewer the complications. Lower blood-glucose levels are found before each meal and at bedtime. Higher blood sugars are found after meals. One hour after a meal, the blood sugar would be higher than two hours after a meal. If a person could remember to test for blood-sugar levels on arising and two hours after a meal, more information for control would be obtained than if the more easily remembered premeal and bedtime blood-sugar tests are used. (Table 9.1 lists the steps for testing blood sugar.) Again, a physician's or other health professional's preference may guide the person into testing one way or another—that is, testing the fasting blood sugar and two hours after each meal, or before meals and at bedtime. If your health professional does not ask you to do blood-sugar tests at home but does them only in the office, be suspicious that you are not receiving the best of care as recommended by the American Diabetes Association and the American Association of Diabetes Educators.

What to Test

Certainly, the blood sugar should be tested if the person feels unusual or ill. Besides the regular testing practices (a minimum of three to four times a day, five to seven days a week for those with Type 1 diabetes; a minimum of four times a day, three days a week for those with Type 2 diabetes; or four times a day, one day a week for those with diet-controlled Type 2 diabetes), other tests should be added as needed. (Remember, it

Table 9.2 Instructions for Testing Urine for Ketones

1. Collect urine in a nonwaxed cup.
2. Dip stick* or strip in urine, or place one drop of urine on tablet.
3. Wait for time requested.
4. Read.
5. Record.

*Sticks or strips may be held in the stream of urine, but be sure the timing is correct.

has been found that the more information you get from more frequent testing, the better you are able to use that information to normalize blood-glucose levels).

If blood-sugar test results are 250 mg/dl (13.8 mmol) or greater, most health professionals would advise that you test the urine for ketones (see Table 9.2). If you are ill, they would usually advise that you test for ketones in the urine even if your blood-sugar levels are not high. If you are preparing to exercise and find blood-sugar levels of 250 mg/dl (13.8 mmol) or greater, you should test for ketones to determine whether or not you should exercise.

Urine testing for glucose is seldom recommended anymore. The major reason is that an elevated or lowered renal threshold (level at which glucose gets through to the urine passed from the body) will give false information. The renal threshold can be determined by emptying the bladder and comparing tested blood against the urine expressed two to three hours afterward. The renal threshold is determined by matching each blood-sugar result with the urine test that follows it (not the urine test taken at the same time as the blood-sugar test). The normal renal threshold is at blood-sugar levels of 160 to 180 mg/dl (8.8 to 10 mmol). Children and pregnant women often run renal thresholds of less than 160 mg/dl (8.8 mmol). Elderly people have a tendency to have renal thresholds greater than 180 mg/dl (10 mmol), and often greater than 200 mg/dl (11.1 mmol). Remember that damage to blood vessels and nerves begins at blood-sugar levels above 150 mg/dl (8.3 mmol).

If blood-glucose tests are unacceptable and the renal-threshold level is known, information from urine glucose tests is at least somewhat helpful. Certainly, such information is better than no information at all. Note that a value obtained from a second passing of urine will measure sugar more nearly representative of what is found in the blood at that time. The first voided test lets the person know what sugar has accumulated over a period of time, and therefore provides a better measure over time. Many times, the second voided urine will contain the same amount of sugar as the first urine specimen (33 percent of the time). While urine testing for sugar has limited value, it could still be useful for small children (although in this day and age, not recommended) who have tender fingers or for those individuals who have normal renal thresholds. Urine testing for sugar is of practically no value in adults, especially in the elderly.

This brings us back to blood-sugar (glucose) testing. The glycosylated hemoglobin test gives the best overall, average determinations of blood-sugar levels for a period of time. The hemoglobin A1 test (upper limits of normals are around 8 to 9 percent) includes the components or parts of A1a, A1b, and A1c, as previously noted. It is found to respond better to more recent increases or decreases in blood-sugar levels than does the more stable component of this test, the hemoglobin A1c (upper level of normal is around 6 to 7 percent).

There are problems with these tests, however. They can be influenced by sickle-cell disease and other abnormalities of hemoglobin (e.g., thalassemia, fetal hemoglobinemia) and by abnormally high or low hematocrits (a low hematocrit reading may result in a falsely low glycosylated hemoglobin A1c; iron deficiency anemia may result in a falsely high glycosylated hemoglobin A1c reading). If home blood-sugar tests over the past two to three months do not seem to match the results of the glycosylated hemoglobin A1c, then be concerned that something else may be occurring (for example, problems with the machine, with the method or accuracy of the testing, or with hemoglobin or hematocrit levels or other abnormal values of the complete blood count [CBC]). Most health professionals prefer to check the hemoglobin A1c every three months.

Also, as noted earlier, fructosamine and glycosylated-serum protein levels demonstrate average blood-sugar levels up to about two to three weeks. The first test measures the glucose levels associated with the albumin in the blood; the second measures the glycosylation that has occurred in the other proteins found in the serum of the blood. The second test is more stable than the first, but it is also more expensive. The upper limit of normal for the fructosamine test is 2.8 percent (280 mg), and for glycosylated protein it is about 8 percent.

Management Approaches

Daily self-monitoring of blood-glucose (SMBG) levels gives the most information. These tests can demonstrate a pattern that may be a reflection of food and medication and of the interactions of these with the person's activity and stressors at home, school, or work. There is a concern about immediately responding to a test result with an increase or decrease of insulin. For a small child, unless he or she is ill and without predicting the activity, the extra dose might send him or her diving into an insulin reaction. Withholding a dose of insulin because the blood-sugar test is in the normal range may start a series of events leading to a "roller-coaster" type of response (also termed "rainbow therapy," meaning that you are always chasing the pot of gold at the end of the rainbow but never catching it!).

The algorithm method of insulin adjustment is at least based on the giving of insulin over and above the usual baseline daily dose. Thus the person is not left in the situation of receiving no insulin and then having to play "catch-up" at a later time. One unit of insulin is usually given for every 50 mg/dl (2.7 mmol) of blood sugar above 150 mg/dl (8.3 mmol). The problem with this approach is that a forty-pound (or 20-kg) child will have a more sensitive response to one unit of insulin than will a 140-pound (or 70-kg) adult.

Unless the person is ill, when supplemental insulin is used to respond to high blood-sugar levels in order to keep the person out of diabetic ketoacidosis, infrequent blood-sugar "spikes" may represent one-time emotional responses and therefore do not require an immediate response. If a pattern develops in the elevation or lowering of blood-sugar levels, something should be done before that blood-sugar response occurs rather than after the fact. Using this approach, health professionals teach people to review their records every two to three days and make adjustments to affect patterns that are observed. Those professionals who use the algorithm approach individualize the amount of insulin to be given when the blood-sugar levels are 150 mg/dl (8.3 mmol) or higher. If this extra insulin is needed frequently, it is added to the previous dose. For the adult, a combination of both of these methods may be successful.

Perhaps clearer explanations of management methods are needed. There are several methods of managing insulin, as follows.

Method 1: Complete Management by the Health Professional

The health professional may or may not have the patient do SMBG. Whatever the testing method(s) used, all data are brought to the health professional, who makes all decisions on changes in insulin and food.

Method 2: Sliding Scale

With this method the patient is allowed to make decisions on changes in insulin based on tables of blood-sugar values and insulin to be injected or withheld. The sliding scale has two major defects. First, insulin is given after the fact—that is, a blood-sugar level at noon, for example, does not predict the insulin needed for the next four to six hours but rather reflects the insulin needed four to six hours ago. You are thus always four to six hours behind and on a roller coaster of control. The other defect is that there is a cutoff point of blood sugar below which no insulin is given. It must be remembered that short-acting insulin lasts only six hours (and rapid-acting insulin only about three hours), so even when there is a low normal blood-sugar level, some insulin must be given to cover the food to be eaten and the time when the previous dose has run out.

Method 3: Algorithms

Algorithms are formulas for changing insulin. They are similar to the sliding scale, except that the formulas are superimposed on a background of two or more doses of intermediate (NPH or lente) or long-acting (ultralente or glargine) insulin. Rapid- or short-acting insulin at mealtimes and/or in the evening is changed on a formula basis, depending on the blood sugar at the time. The major defect of this system is that the rapid- or short-acting insulin is again given after the fact. The system can be made to work, however, by choosing the amount of supplemental insulin based on changes in the food intake or activity levels or on the consistent need to add extra insulin to the previous dose.

An example of the latter management is as follows: Suppose a person is taking a mixture of NPH and regular for breakfast, with regular for supper and NPH at bedtime, and he or she has persistently high blood-sugar levels before breakfast. This person has an algorithm to increase the morning regular insulin by one unit for every 50 mg that the blood sugar is above 150 mg/dl (8.3 mmol), and would thus increase the morning regular if this elevated blood sugar occurred. However, the problem of the increased fasting blood sugar means there is a need for more NPH at bedtime, not for more regular insulin in the morning. An increase in morning regular may cause a reaction later in the morning. If the algorithm is used, the extra regular insulin given in the morning should be called supplemental insulin and recorded in the logbook separately. If the problem is recurrent (several days in a row), then the "supplement" should be added by increasing the evening NPH rather than by taking the regular continually as a morning supplement.

Method 4: Patterned Glucose Approach

In this method, a basic two-, three-, four-, or more-dose insulin regimen is prescribed, and blood sugar is tested four times (either fasting and two hours after each meal, or premeal and at bedtime) for three consecutive days. The pattern of blood-sugar values is then analyzed, and the appropriate insulin or insulins are altered prior to the time of altered blood-sugar levels. Example: The person is taking NPH/regular before breakfast, regular before supper, and NPH at bedtime. The blood sugar is tested before breakfast and after breakfast or prelunch, after lunch or presupper, and after supper or at bedtime. A target range of blood-sugar values for each time period is prescribed, and the achieved values over the three-day period are compared with the target.

If the prebreakfast blood-sugar level is too high or too low (our acceptable target is 60 to 120 mg/dl [3.3 to 6.6 mmol]), the NPH, lente, or Lantus given at bedtime is changed. If the level after breakfast or prelunch is outside the target range (70 to 150 mg/dl [3.8 to 8.3 mmol]), then the morning regular, Novolog, or Humalog is changed. If the afternoon blood sugar is off (range desired is 70 to 150 mg/dl [3.8 to 8.3 mmol]), then the morning NPH, lente, or split Lantus is changed. If the evening or bedtime blood sugar is out of range (70 to 150 mg/dl [3.8 to 8.3 mmol]), then the supper regular, Novolog, or Humalog insulin is changed.

Method 5: Advanced Patterned Management

As you become more familiar with how much insulin is needed for how much food in relation to what level of activity, you can use this predictive approach safely. Again, this approach does not react to the current blood-glucose levels but rather predicts how much insulin will be needed in relation to what food is to be eaten and what activity is planned for later that day, especially if it requires heavy work or play. There is a guideline termed the "1,500 Rule" (alternatively called the 1,800 Rule) often used by people on insulin infusion pumps or as a starting number to address how much insulin is needed for each carbohydrate or calorie counted. The 1,500 Rule is calculated as follows: 1,500 (or 1,800) divided by the total number of units of insulin in one day equals the insulin sensitivity. This result multiplied by 0.33 gives the grams of carbohydrate covered by one unit of insulin.

For adults, little calculation is needed. Unless the person is highly sensitive to rapid- or short-acting insulin, the starting point is one unit of insulin for one calorie point (75 calories equal one point). People who use this formula with carbohydrates often use one unit for each CHO (carbohydrate) point (15 g of carbohydrate).

You could take your usual premeal rapid-acting insulin dose and a known amount of carbohydrates or calorie points and check your blood sugar two hours later. Once the two-hour blood sugars are in an acceptable range, increase or decrease the premeal insulin to get the desired postmeal glucose response, then divide the insulin by the food to get the food insulin ratio for that meal. Example: Six units of insulin result in a two-hour aftermeal blood sugar of 120 mg/dl when six points of food are eaten with usual activity. The food/insulin ratio is one unit of insulin per one point of food (75 calories).

Note: It is recommended that the bedtime blood sugar be around 100 mg/dl (5.5 mmol); the range for small children should be higher but not greater than 180 mg/dl (10 mmol), unless Lantus is used.

If a different insulin regimen is used, the same principles apply. Just remember that the therapeutic (or pharmacodynamic) action of rapid- and short-acting, intermediate, and long-acting insulins are shorter in duration than the zero insulin levels to zero insulin levels (pharmacokinetic responses) found in the package inserts.

By understanding when a given insulin peaks and what its duration is, you will know when to check your blood sugar and how to use the results to change the insulin dose. Hemoglobin A1c's less than 7 percent, or even less than 6.5 percent, may be safely achieved.

Testing Supplies and Equipment

A number of supplies are needed for home testing of blood-sugar levels: lancets to pierce the finger, the finger-piercing device or arm-piercing device, and the machine and/or sticks or tablets used to test blood or urine. The most effective way to clean the fingers is by washing the hands with soap and warm water. Traveling? Alcohol or other cleansing wipes are useful to have on hand.

Urine Tests

Tests for glucose in the urine are the tablet test (Clinitest) and the stick test (Clinistix Strips and Diastix). The tests for ketones are the tablet test (Acetest) and the stick test (Chemstrip K and Ketostix strips, also available in individual foil-wrapped packets). Combination tests that test for glucose and ketones are Chemstrip uGK and Keto-Diastix. Biotel is available for various screening tests of the urine, as are Multichem strips. Micral test strips are available to check for small amounts of protein in the urine (microalbuminuria).

Lancets

Lancets should be sharp and easy to hold (by hand or by machine). Some lancets fit some machines but not others. These include the Accu-Chek Softclix and Soft Touch, BD Ultra-Fine II Lancets, ComforTouch Unilet, E-Z Ject, Gentle-let, Haemolance, Lady Lite and Lite Touch, Medi-Lance and Medi-Lance II, Microlet, Monolet Original and Thin, OneTouch, Prestige, ReliOn, Techlite, Tenderlett, Tenderlett Jr, and Tenderlett Toddler. There are also the Unilet and Vitalet Lancets. (Refer to the *Diabetes Forecast Resource Guide*, published one or more times a year by the American Diabetes Association, for more information on these lancets, to find out whether the points are beveled or fine, and to learn whether these lancets fit all lancing devices or not.)

Lancing devices that hold the lancets are also becoming more numerous and varied. The pen-shaped devices are the Monoject, Penlet II, Gentle-Lance Lancet Device, and Select Lite Lancing Device. The BD Lancet Device has specially designed 30-gauge BD Ultra-Fine II Lancets. The Autolet Mini, Autolet Clinisafe, and the Autolet Lite have platforms that control the depth of penetration. The Accu-Chek Softclix Lancet Device has eleven depth settings (see Figure 9.1).

A number of devices now on the market are able to get blood from an arm or the side of the hand. Vaculance is a device with a vacuumlike action that is able to pull blood to the surface from any part of the body. There is some controversy in relation to the delay in getting the blood-sugar reading from the blood from the arm versus the finger. It is recommended to rub the target site on the arm before obtaining a blood sample.

There are so many lancing devices (e.g., Gentle-lance Lancet Device, Lite Touch Lancing Device, Monojector Lancet Device, Personal Lasette Laser Lancing Device, Prestige Lite Touch Lancing Device, and Ultra TLC Adjustable Lancing Device, to name a few) and lancets available that space does not allow us to list them all. New ones will become available between the writing and printing of this book. We suggest the following guidelines for selecting this equipment:

1. Check with your pharmacist and try some of the devices to see which one works best for you.
2. Check the *ADA Forecast* magazine. This excellent monthly publication from the ADA contains much useful material. The most useful tool is the *Resource Guide* published one or more times a year, which is devoted to supplies and equipment.

Continual upgrading and improvements have been done on the lancets, strips, and machines for measuring blood-sugar levels.

Figure 9.1 Lancing Devices

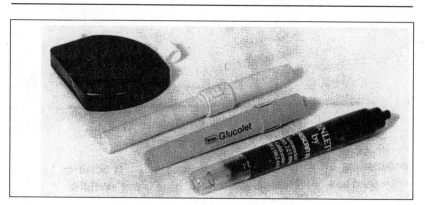

The quality of the instruments, lancets, and strips continues to be high, and technology is improving almost daily.

Sticks

Sight-reading blood-glucose test strips is much less accurate but may be used as a quick check when a machine is not available. The strip specifically designed for sight-reading is the BG Chemstrip. This test strip has a two-minute timing unless the blood-glucose reading is 240 mg/dl (13.3 mmol) or higher. If it is higher, then an extra minute is needed to sight-read the final results. The two color areas for each blood-glucose determination (i.e., 40 or 80 or 120) give room for some interpretation of potential midpoints between the numbers (i.e., 60 or 100, etc.).

Machines

Blood-glucose monitors are very helpful. Rebates, trade-ins, and specials made available by the manufacturers to pharmacies and clinics make the monitors very inexpensive or, in some cases, even free.

Roche Diagnostics makes several meters (see Figure 9.2). They include the Accu-Chek Advantage, the Accu-Chek Softclix, the Accu-Chek Active (five-second test), and the Accu-Chek Compact (the meter holds a "drum" of seventeen strips). The Accu-Chek Complete is the most sophisticated. It holds a variety of information for times and

Figure 9.2 Examples of Blood-Glucose Monitors

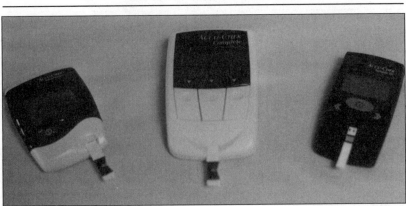

Figure 9.3 Accu-Chek Equipment for Downloading and Printing Blood-Sugar Tests

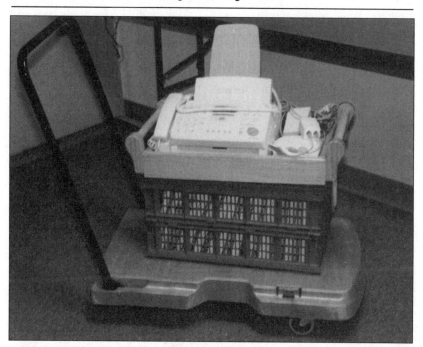

values for blood sugar (1,000 tests) and can also record other information such as the time and dose of the insulin. It can be connected to a computer and with the appropriate software supplied by the company (Accu-Chek Compass) can be off-loaded. The computer can then analyze the data and print out logbooks, graphs, and other helpful materials for easy evaluation of where the problems are and the changes needed in the program to correct the problems (see Figure 9.3). This company also has a strip that is curved on the side to allow the finger to easily fit against the strip to obtain the blood (Comfort Curve strips take only twenty-five seconds to get results). This system takes less blood and is simpler to use than the strips that require blood on the top of the strip. The Advantage and Complete may also be off-loaded, by modem, to a fax machine and the results faxed to a clinic.

Bayer Corporation's (now under the name of Ascencia) most popular machines are the Glucometer Elite, which has a thirty-second test, the Glucometer EliteXL, and the Glucometer DEX2, which has a fifteen- to sixty-second test, depending on the height of the blood-glucose value. Both have a ten-test memory, and both read up to 500 or higher. The capillary action of the Elite is an added advantage to those who aren't able to get much blood from a finger or have difficulty getting the drop on the strip.

Home Diagnostics makes two meters that give results in ten to fifty seconds (both have memories for 365 tests): PrestigeLX and PrestigeIQ. Both use plasma or whole blood. Lifescan, Inc., presently has several popular machines: the OneTouch Basic, OneTouch Ultra, OneTouch Profile, and Sure Step. All read from zero to 500 or higher. OneTouch Basic gives the previous test result. The Basic and Profile test whole blood while the other machine reads in plasma levels. The Profile stores 250 tests and averages out the tests done at various times of the day, and the Sure Step stores ten tests. All the OneTouch machines take forty-five seconds. The Sure Step takes fifteen to thirty seconds and requires only a small blood sample. The OneTouch II, OneTouch Profile, OneTouch Ultra (a five-second test), and OneTouch Ultra Smart can also be connected to a computer and off-loaded. The software can then analyze the data and print it out in various forms, including a logbook format and various kinds of graphs.

Abbott Laboratories also makes several meters: the Precision Xtra, Precision QID, and Sof-Tact. The Precision Xtra and the Sof-Tact hold 450 readings. The Precision QID holds ten readings. Each has an associated computer program similar to the ones described above. These meters use a strip that uses capillary action and thus needs very little blood.

TheraSense makes the FreeStyle Meter (250 test memory; reaction time five to fifteen seconds). This meter is capable of testing blood from and including sites other than the fingertips. (FreeStyle, OneTouch Ultra, and Sof-Tact are FDA-approved for alternate site testing.) The FreeStyle meter also has the FreeStyle Tracker, a hand-held meter and computer combined.

There are some meter and strip limitations, such as ease of use and quality of the product, that are being addressed by various companies. These companies are continuing to improve the strips in relation to response to humidity, temperature, and altitude. Individuals with impaired vision have some problems "hitting the target" or getting the drop of blood directly on the place provided on the strip. The Elite and the Sure Step help overcome this barrier to testing. Sound units (e.g., OneTouch II and Freedom) allow the visually impaired to have a sense of independence with audible, user friendly devices that may be attached to their standard machines. Diascan is a familiar older machine and one of the first to address the problems of sight.

Data managers off-load the information from the blood-glucose monitors and put it in a desired format, such as a graph or printout. More sophisticated systems use a meter that can store nearly 3,000 events (such as blood sugar, insulin dose, food intake, exercise, and so forth).

Testing is a necessary part of monitoring daily care. Choosing products carefully makes daily care easier. Product quality has proved to be stable throughout the spectrum of those on the market. Any product that has been found to be below standard has been immediately recalled by the company for alteration and upgrading.

This is not an exhaustive list of available meters but only a list of the most commonly used ones (see Table 9.3). Several others are available and new ones are being developed to replace the older models and their strips. Check with your pharmacist or your diabetes educator for the meter that best meets your needs, and check out the *ADA Forecast* magazine or *Diabetes Self-Management* for frequent updates. Also, check with your insurance company. Some companies, particularly the HMOs, may have contracts with a specific company and carry only one type of strip. You may also find some generic models available in stores such as Wal-Mart and Kmart.

Check before you buy. You do not want to get a meter, even a free one, and then find that your insurance company will not pay for strips for that machine. Your diabetes educator is one of the best people to help you with these problems and help you get the very best machine for your particular needs.

Bloodless sugar testing will one day be a reality. Even as this book goes to press, new machines that are easier to use, lighter, and less expensive will likely become available. Wishful thinking? Not necessarily. Such a machine is being developed today. And although it will be a while before such machines can be made small enough or inexpensive enough for home use, take time to remember that computers once took up whole rooms and cost a fortune but are now small enough to fit into a pocket or purse.

Table 9.3 Blood-Glucose Meters

Meter	Range	Test Time (Seconds)
ACCU-CHEK "Advantage"	10–600	40
ACCU-CHEK "Complete"	10–600	40
ACCU-CHEK "Active"	10–600	5
ACCU-CHEK "Compact"	10–600	15
ACCU-CHEK "Voicemate"	10–600	26
Produced by Roche Diagnostics (800) 858-8072		
BD Logic	20–600	5
BD Latitude	20–600	5
Produced by Becton, Dickinson and Co. (BD) (888) 232-2737		
"FreeStyle"	20–500	15
Produced by TheraSense (888) 522-5226		
GLUCOMETER "Dex" and "Dex 2"	10–600	30
GLUCOMETER "Elite"	20–600	30
GLUCOMETER "Elite XL"	20–600	30
Distributed by Bayer Diagnostics under the name of Ascencia (800) 348-8100		
ONETOUCH "Basic"	0–600	45
ONETOUCH "New Basic"	0–600	45
ONETOUCH "Profile"	0–600	45
ONETOUCH "Sure Step"	0–500	15–30
ONETOUCH "Ultra"	20–600	5
ONETOUCH "Ultra Smart"	20–600	5
ONETOUCH "In Duo"	20–600	5
Produced by Lifescan, Inc. (800) 227-8862		
PRECISION "QID"	20–600	20
PRECISION "Xtra"	20–600	20 for glucose 30 for ketones
PRECISION "Sof-Tact"	30–450	20
Produced by Medisense, Inc. (800) 527-3339		
PRESTIGE LX	25–600	5 to 50
PRESTIGE IQ	25–600	5 to 50

Produced by Home Diagnostics (cobranded by Medicine Shoppe, Walgreens, Osco, K-Mart, Albertsons, CVS, Publix, and Wynn Dixie. Called the "Prestige Smart System" (800) 342-7226

Summary

Self-monitoring of blood glucose, the greatest innovation in diabetes care in the past fifteen years, now allows us to attain the degree of control necessary to prevent the serious complications of the disease. Every person with diabetes mellitus, whether Type 1 or Type 2, should be doing self-testing. When diabetes is unstable (such as in illness) or when changes are being made, the testing should be carried out four times or more per day, every day. When diabetes mellitus is stable, less testing is necessary but is still encouraged.

We feel, from extensive experience, that it is necessary for persons with Type 1 diabetes to do self-testing of blood sugar (SMBG) four times a day for a minimum of five days a week. For persons with Type 2 diabetes, it is necessary to monitor four times per day, at least three days a week unless the person is diet controlled (then once a week is adequate unless the person is ill). For persons taking insulin, whether they have Type 1 or Type 2, it is necessary to have a machine to do SMBG. For persons with Type 2 who are using diet alone or diet plus oral agents, testing with a visual strip is permissible, but machine testing is encouraged.

The data obtained from self-monitoring of blood glucose allow frequent responses through adjustments in the food and diabetes medication in relation to activity. Combined with spaced measurements of hemoglobin A1c, fructosamine, or glycosylated proteins, self-testing is extremely effective in facilitating and supporting blood sugar control.

Now, even hemoglobin A1c testing (the percentage of glucose attached to protein in the red blood cells over two to three months) may be done at home (about $15 per test.) Called A1cNow (www.rx4betterhealth.com) or In Charge (produced by LXN, it measures glucose and fructosamine), the tests indicate the average of continuous glucose changes over the previous two to three weeks. These tests give overall information but do not indicate where the problem might be (e.g., hypoglycemia or hyperglycemia frequencies). They are helpful in that they include the times you are not testing, but they do not take the place of daily or every other day monitoring (four or so times a day).

It bears repeating: With good control you will feel better and be more energetic and more productive. Most important, you will be in control of your own life and destiny and will therefore be better able to prevent both acute, intermediate, and chronic complications of the disease.

10

What Are the Possible Complications of Diabetes?

Any time the body chemistry is out of balance, there are bound to be adverse changes in body tissue. The environment, the things you eat, the stresses you are under, and whatever illnesses or disabilities you may be fighting all make a difference in the physiological functioning of your body (that is, the way your body responds). If you have a way to control the "stimulators" of these changes, it will be possible for you to minimize the damage that such changes can cause. So it is with diabetes mellitus. The body cells are accustomed to only so much glucose in the system. If there is too much or too little, changes take place in cell function, size, and structure.

There are three series of changes that occur with the person who has diabetes: acute changes, intermediate changes, and chronic changes. Acute changes, or complications, are diabetic ketoacidosis, hypoglycemia, and hyperglycemic hyperosmolar nonketotic syndrome. Intermediate complications are those involving illness, surgery, pregnancy, and travel. Chronic complications involve the nerves (neuropathy), the kidneys (nephropathy), the eyes (retinopathy), and macroangiopathy of the heart and large blood vessels (cardiomyopathy: peripheral, cerebral, and cardiovascular). Chronic complications are noticeable by pain, numbness, inability to see, inability to go to the bathroom, and inability to otherwise function. Retinopathy, nephropathy, neuropathy, and cardiomyopathy have association, directly or indirectly, with small blood vessels.

Acute Complications

Diabetic Ketoacidosis

Diabetic ketoacidosis is preceded by diabetic ketosis, which itself is preceded by hyperglycemia. As already discussed, hyperglycemia can occur when there is an absolute lack or relative unavailability of insulin. Diabetic ketosis occurs when insulin is deficient and glucose is no longer able to get into the cells. When this occurs, an alternate source of energy is needed. The result is the production of ketone bodies from free fatty acids. Diabetic ketoacidosis, the most severe state, occurs when an imbalance due to a severe or prolonged insulin deficiency leads to dehydration and a chemical (electrolyte) imbalance. (See Table 10.1 for signs and symptoms of diabetic ketoacidosis.)

Diabetic ketoacidosis is a serious condition. The blood-glucose levels are not necessarily extremely high (for example, in the case of an infant, the blood glucose value could be 190 mg/dl [10.5 mmol]). Usually, however, the level is in the range of 300 to 900 mg/dl (16.6 to 50 mmol). The production of ketones from the fat breakdown makes the body more acidic. This is when the acute problem occurs, since the body cannot exist if it is too acid or too alkaline. Acidity is manifested or noted by chemistry (biochemically) and by labored breathing (Kussmaul, or heavy and labored respirations). Kussmaul respiration is the body's attempt to break down and blow off some of the acid in the system (carbon dioxide and its earlier form, carbonic acid).

Diabetic ketoacidosis is treated with intravenous fluids (to dilute the glucose levels in the system and rehydrate the dehydrated person), with insulin (to aid in helping glucose get into the cells), and with chemicals called electrolytes (usually potassium, sodium, phosphates, and bicarbonates). Two of the most common chemicals needing replacement are potassium and sodium. These are involved in cellular functions related to electrical changes in the body, particularly in the heart and the brain. The first fluids given are called "plasma expanders," which can be anything from blood to saline. Normal saline (a body-balanced salt-and-water solution) is usually the fluid of choice.

Once the blood-glucose levels drop to a certain point (that is, about 300 mg/dl [17 mmol]), the body needs some fuel so that it will not

Table 10.1 Diabetic Ketoacidosis from Hyperglycemia

	Signs and Symptoms	Causes	Treatments
Hyperglycemia	Increased thirst Increased urination	Not enough insulin, not enough exercise, too much food, stress, medications	Fluids, insulin
Glucosuria	Dehydration Blurry vision	Growth, pregnancy, illness	Fluids, insulin
Ketosis	Fruity breath Weight loss Acetone in urine Blood sugars usually over 250 mg/dl (13.8 mmol)		Fluids, insulin Fluids, insulin
Ketoacidosis	Electroyte imbalance Nausea Vomiting Kussmaul respiration Pulse fast and "thready" (i.e., thin, weak)		Fluids, insulin, potassium, other chemicals as needed
Coma	The most severe state of DKA		Fluids, insulin, potassium, other chemicals as needed
Hyperosmolar Nonketotic Syndrome*	No coma, dehydration	Dehydration, hyperglycemia	Fluids, potassium, little insulin

*Seldom seen in Type 1 Diabetes

call on more ketones (ketogenesis) for energy and hypoglycemia will not occur. Glucose is added as part of the saline solution (D5 or D10 usually in half of normal saline). The choice depends on whether there is a balance in the saline level in the body, as determined (analyzed) by frequent electrolyte analyses by the lab. Potassium is almost always added to the intravenous fluids, as are other chemicals, if such chemicals do not rebalance in the rehydration process. Insulin is also given, usually intravenously, until the blood-glucose levels are near normal and more stable.

Hypoglycemia

Hypoglycemia can be separated into the true low-blood-glucose state or the "false" state that mimics low-blood-glucose-level responses. Adrenaline is released when the body feels it is in crisis, resulting in the symptoms of shakiness, trembling, irritability, hunger, and weakness.

"False" hypoglycemia occurs when blood-glucose levels are not below normal range but drop rapidly over a short period of time, or when blood-glucose levels are at a point that the body is unaccustomed to. If the person has had very high blood-glucose levels for a long period of time and treatment allows the blood sugar to be at a more normal level, symptoms of hypoglycemia may occur. A blood-glucose level of 50 to 80 mg/dl (2.7 to 4.4 mmol), depending on the individual's physiological awareness, or a fall in the glucose level of 100 mg/dl (5.5 mmol) in a short period of time can cause the symptoms of low blood sugar. The symptoms are those of adrenaline release, not of true below-normal glucose levels or of hypoglycemia. (See Table 10.2 for signs and symptoms of hypoglycemia.)

True hypoglycemia occurs when blood-glucose levels fall below the normal range (that is, less than 60 mg/dl [3.3 mmol] for whole blood). Hunger, some irritability, and perhaps a little weakness occurs when the levels are 40 to 60 mg/dl (2.2 to 3.3 mmol) (Level I). At 20 to 40 mg/dl (1.1 to 2.2 mmol) (Level II), dilated pupils, trembling, sweating, and a stronger, more rapid pulse rate occur (remember, this type of pulse rate indicates only that adrenaline has been released and so can also occur with false hypoglycemia). Unconsciousness, seizurelike activity, or other neurological manifestations are seen when blood-glucose levels are below 20 mg/dl (1.1 mmol) (Level III).

Symptoms are different from person to person. If a person has had Type 1 diabetes for a long period of time (that is, five years or longer), it is possible that the symptoms may change. Some specialists feel that in such a case the body has become "overchallenged" through the years. Whatever stimulated the release of adrenaline before is now ignored, and the body blunts or changes its warning symptoms.

As noted earlier in this book, food in small amounts is often all that is needed for Level I hypoglycemia. Level II usually requires some simple sugar to bring the blood-glucose level up to 40 mg/dl (2.2 mmol) and higher to relieve symptoms. Food will usually be used properly at blood-glucose levels greater than 40 mg/dl (2 mmol).

Level III requires 50 percent glucose, glucagon (see Figure 10.1), or some thick liquid glucose product (for example, honey), placed either inside the cheek or under the tongue. If a person is having seizurelike activity, it would not be safe to give oral glucose, since it could be inhaled into the lungs. At home, a injection of glucagon into muscle tissue is the preferred treatment. (Note: If glucagon is used, simple sugars are given to replace glycogen stores and to overcome nausea when the person arouses; food can be given after the person is no longer nauseated.) Every insulin-taking person with diabetes should have glucagon available at home, at school, at work, and when traveling. (Note:

Table 10.2 Insulin Reaction—Hypoglycemia, Insulin Shock

Level	Symptoms	Treatment
Mild: I	Irritable, trembly, weak, shaky, hungry. Blood sugar 41–60 mg/dl (2.3–3.3 mmol)	Food (general snack— carbohydrate and protein)* Food or drink (one-half to one calorie point in milk, or a snack with protein and carbohydrate). Next regular meal or snack as scheduled, then rest for 15 minutes. Contact a health professional.
Moderate: II	Skin cold and clammy to the touch; pale face; shallow, fast breathing; drowsy Blood sugar 21–40 mg/dl (1.2–2.2 mmol)	Simple sugar (20–40 calories); small snack 10–15 minutes later; then 15 minutes of rest.
Severe: III	Unconscious, possible convulsions, danger of swallowing incorrectly Protect person by placing on side or stomach, and keep airway open. Blood sugar usually less than 20 mg/dl (1.1 mmol)	Glucagon injection; simple sugar; food with protein 15–20 minutes later. Notify physician.

Wear Medic Alert Bracelet!

CAUSES OF INSULIN REACTION
- Unusual physical exertion or exercise without increasing food or decreasing insulin
- An overdose of insulin or pills due to a mistake in measuring
- Mistake in the meal plan
- Failure to reduce insulin after an infection
- Poor usage of the meal due to vomiting or diarrhea
- Delay in eating a meal or snack

*Important note: If blood sugars are low at injection time, be sure to treat until the blood sugar is up to 100 mg/dl (5.5 mmol), then take injection and have something to eat immediately.

Dosages for glucagon are 0.25 mg for children three years of age and younger; 0.5 mg for children three to five years old; and 1 mg for anyone older than five.)

Hyperglycemic Hyperosmolar Nonketotic Syndrome

This syndrome is a subtle but quite severe hyperglycemic episode in which the acid state (ketoacidosis) does not develop but dehydration is very acute. This condition is now more frequently called a syndrome rather than a coma, because the majority of people are diagnosed before they ever reach the state of coma. Blood-glucose levels may be in the neighborhood of 800 to 2,000 mg/dl (44.4 to 111.1 mmol). Osmolarity is the level of water concentration, or dehydration, of the body. The higher it is, the worse the outcome for the person involved. Dehydration must be attended to first; insulin is then given in carefully prescribed doses, as individuals with this condition are very insulin sensitive.

In diabetic ketoacidosis there are ketones in the blood and urine. In hyperglycemic hyperosmolar nonketotic syndrome, there are few, if any, ketones in the blood and urine, because the person is making just enough insulin or using oral medication to suppress ketogenesis (the making of new ketones) but not enough to control the sugar. The large amount of fluid lost also means the loss of much potassium. Replacement of potassium is done during the acute state and usually for some time afterward. The more potassium lost and the greater the state of dehydration of the person, the greater the seriousness of the illness.

Intermediate Complications

Intermediate complications are those that involve various stressors such as illness, emotional upset, surgery, pregnancy, and travel.

Complications Due to Illness and Stress

More insulin is required during most illnesses. A few illnesses, such as those with vomiting and diarrhea, require either less insulin or a delay in insulin administration. The usual response to high fever is higher

Figure 10.1 Glucagon Emergency Kit

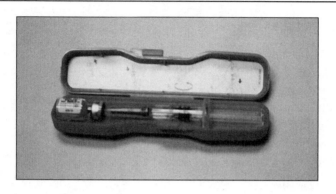

blood-glucose levels. The more ill or dehydrated the person becomes, the higher the blood-glucose levels will be. The object in dealing with the illness is to keep the diabetes out of the picture (i.e., the illness acts as a stressor that could cause the person to go into diabetic ketoacidosis; if the diabetes is adequately treated, then only the illness needs to be the focus of treatment). If the medication taken is in a sugar solution or in some other way elevates blood-glucose levels, the insulin should be raised to cover it. If the person is on an oral agent or on a diet alone program, insulin may be required during the acute phase of the illness.

Prevention is, of course, best (for example, getting flu shots and keeping immunizations up to date). If an illness does occur, vigorous treatment is needed. If the illness or treatment causes the blood-glucose levels to go up, increased insulin is needed. (Note: Prolonged emotional stress will act just like an illness on the body, so treatment needs to be the same. The higher the blood-glucose levels, the more insulin is needed, depending on ketone levels.)

Whether you have Type 1 or Type 2 diabetes, it is important during illness or stress to monitor your blood-glucose levels carefully and frequently, and to know when to notify your health professional. Your health care team should give you some rules for what to eat and drink at these times and how to supplement your insulin doses or alter your oral agent. To make these changes in medication, however, you need to know your blood-glucose values. If you have these data, it is a simple matter of mathematics to respond appropriately and to prevent diabetic ketoacidosis or hyperglycemic hyperosmolar nonketotic syndrome.

Complications Due to Surgery

Surgery, whether for a minor or a major problem, is also a stressor to the body. If the person is on an oral agent, the physician may request that the agent be discontinued for a period of time before, during, and after the surgery, and insulin substituted for treatment.

If the person has Type 1 diabetes, normalization of blood-glucose levels prior to, during, and after surgery will help speed up the healing process. If the blood-glucose levels are elevated, there is a decrease in fibroblasts (the cells that heal wounds) and a decrease in available white blood cells, with the result being a greater chance of infection. (Note: If scientists want germs to grow on an agar plate, they add one thing—glucose.) Many specialists are recognizing that some insulin is needed. It may be given in a small amount without food, or in a somewhat larger amount when the intravenous fluids are begun in preparation for the surgical procedure, during the procedure, and for a short while afterward.

Complications with Pregnancy

If the blood-glucose levels are kept normal from preconception or the prepregnancy state through delivery, the chances of having a normal baby are the same for a diabetic woman as they are for a nondiabetic woman. If the blood-glucose levels are not controlled during the first trimester of pregnancy (the first three months), there is a 14 percent chance of congenital malformations, fetal loss, or maternal complications. The goal is to maintain the blood-glucose levels in the range of 60 to 90 mg/dl (3.3 to 5.0 mmol) fasting, and 70 to 120 mg/dl (3.8 to 6.6 mmol) two hours after a meal. This is true for women with gestational diabetes (diabetes just during pregnancy) as well as for women with fully diagnosed Type 1 or Type 2 diabetes. If a woman has been on oral agents, she must be started on insulin preferably before pregnancy because of the potential side effects of oral agents on the fetus. If a pregnant woman has difficulty controlling blood-glucose levels, insulin is given via an infusion pump or in four or more doses of short or rapid-acting insulin per day.

Insulin needs generally increase during the nine months, especially as caloric needs increase (often 300 calories above baseline during the last trimester). Once the baby is delivered, the need for insulin decreases even if the mother is nursing the infant (mother's food needs are usually 500 calories above baseline during this time). Women with gestational diabetes often need to stop insulin, while those with Type 1 diabetes need less insulin and those with Type 2 diabetes return to the use of an oral agent(s).

Complications During Travel

Much preplanning must be done so that travel, whether for pleasure or for business, is a safe and rewarding experience. If you are going overseas, some names and numbers to know are as follows: Centers for Disease Control International Travelers Hotline: 1-800-311-3435; International Association for Medical Assistance to Travelers: (716) 754-4883; Traveler Assistance International: 1-800-821-2828; Travelers Emergency Network: 1-800-275-4836; and Travelex Insurance Services, Inc.: 1-800-228-9792. These organizations can give you the names of doctors in other countries who know about diabetes management. They can also tell you what supplies are available in other countries and how to ask for assistance in other languages.

If you will be crossing more than two time zones, many specialists advise you to change to multiple doses of short- or rapid-acting insulin. The rapid-acting insulin is most convenient as it may be given just before meals (usually every four hours on an overseas flight). An insulin-infusion pump or baseline insulins (e.g., NPH, ultralente, glargine) work very well for travel since they allow for a basal insulin, while a bolus insulin (e.g., lispro, aspart) may be given right with the meal. It is usually recommended that you stay on multiple doses for twenty-four to forty-eight hours after you reach your destination.

The two cardinal rules for travel: Always keep your insulin with you (not in your suitcase), and always keep some food handy.

Chronic Complications

Chronic complications are perhaps the most feared, even though when they are caught early there is a chance of reversing some of the processes.

It is only when there is an end-stage process working (that is, when there has been cell damage or destruction) that little can be done. Again: The best way to prevent or delay complications is to keep the blood-glucose levels in the normal range as much of the time as possible, without the occurrence of any significant insulin reactions.

Neuropathy

Neuropathy is easily recognized by burning and tingling sensations, pain or numbness, and lack of function. The pain associated with neuropathy often decreases with lowered and normalized blood-glucose levels, but it may even increase temporarily as nerves and nerve endings are replaced. The discomfort of neuropathy may be worse at night, and you may feel some discomfort from the bedclothes touching your feet (an object can be placed on the bed, with the covers placed over it so that they do not touch your feet). No one knows why the discomfort increases at night, but it is possible that it is simply increased perception of pain when there is nothing else to distract your attention.

Pain may also increase during the healing process. Perhaps as new blood vessels form and as the nerves become resensitized or new ones grow, they initially are more sensitive. The increased discomfort may thus mean that something is improving rather than that something is wrong. Your physician or other health care professional will assist you so that you can be as comfortable as possible during this potentially uncomfortable time (the discomfort usually lasts about six months to a year).

Some people feel more discomfort with exercise, even with just mild walking. This discomfort may not be related to neuropathy alone. Pain in the legs with walking that is relieved by rest is probably due to an obstruction to blood flow in an artery of the leg due to diabetes or general vascular (blood vessel) disease (that is, you can have high cholesterol levels but not have diabetes). This cramping condition is called "intermittent claudication." Medications may be given that allow the blood to flow more freely through the blood vessels. Another treatment is to open an artery through angioplasty (a balloon) or laser treatment, or through surgically bypassing the obstruction (bypass graft).

Numbness is the other side of the coin. As noted in an earlier chapter, people have experienced bizarre episodes such as having a tack in the foot without knowing it until they do their daily foot inspection!

This is why daily foot inspection is so important (along with not going barefoot). There is less of a chance of reversibility of the nerve damage when numbness is experienced. Some people, is spite of numbness, experience improvement of sensation with the use of alpha lipoic acid, a complementary treatment that affects nerve nutrition.

There are five different types of neuropathy (see Table 10.3).

Distal Symmetrical Polyneuropathy

This type of neuropathy, also called simply polyneuropathy, involves the feet and legs and is usually described by the person as numbness or tingling in the feet. Sometimes a burning sensation is noted. Normalizing blood-glucose levels is the best treatment at present. There are several medications that can help this problem, although none will cure it. Of course pain medications and narcotics will control the pain, but they have

Table 10.3 Diabetes Neuropathies

Distal Symmetrical Polyneuropathy (reversible)	Disease of the end of the nerve	Sensory loss or weakness of hands and feet, absent reflex
Autonomic Neuropathy (treatable, but not easily reversed)	Disease of part of the nervous system that controls automatic body functions (such as the heart, glands, or intestines)	Gastropathy (disease of the stomach, also called gastroparesis), sexual dysfunction, diabetic diarrhea, lack of sweating or increased sweating, stopping of heart or of breathing, postural hypotension (i.e., feeling lightheaded when quickly changing from a lying to a sitting or standing position)
Proximal Motor Neuropathy (reversible)	Disease of the end of the nerve	Weakness and loss of nerves to muscles in hands, thighs, and pelvic area
Cranial Mononeuropathy (reversible)	Disease of spine and cranial (head) nerves	Pain, weakness, sensory loss, or change in reflexes
Radiculopathy (reversible)	Disease of beginnings (roots) of spinal nerves	Pain or sensory loss in an area of the skin

long-term problems. Antidepressants are sometimes helpful as are some antiseizure drugs such as Tegretol and Neurontin. Capsaicin, a derivative of jalipeño peppers, in a cream form, can be helpful in relieving the surface pain and burning. It must be used carefully, that is, be sure to follow the directions and to wash your hands after applying the cream.

Autonomic Neuropathy

This type of neuropathy involves nerves that work without your needing to pay attention to them—for example, nerves relating to control of the blood pressure (orthostatic hypertension), to the stomach or gastrointestinal tract (possible problems include disease of the stomach, called gastroparesis, or the intestine, called diabetic diarrhea), to the sweat glands (loss of the ability to perspire), to the bladder (problems with urinating), to balance, to sexual function, and to the cardiovascular system. Autonomic neuropathy is not as closely associated with diabetes control as is peripheral neuropathy (neuropathy of the hands and feet), but diabetes control is still needed.

There are a variety of treatments that can control the results of autonomic neuropathy. Again, prevention is best. The use of the Anscore machine assists in determining if autonomic neuropathy, concerning the heart and respiration, is present in the body (see Figure 10.2). This test takes about fifteen minutes and prints out a reading that is interpreted for you by the health professional.

Proximal Motor Neuropathy

Also know as diabetic amyotrophy, this type of neuropathy involves damage to the nerves in the muscles, resulting in weakness and shrinking of the muscle fibers. A burning sensation may also be experienced. The hands (especially between the thumb and index finger) and inner thighs are most commonly affected. The ankle joints may also be involved. Resolution or recovery may be experienced in six to eighteen months.

Cranial Mononeuropathy

This type of neuropathy most often involves the eye muscles. Double vision may be present, the eyelids may droop, and the eyes may have problems with drainage. Plain "mononeuropathy" may also involve the

Figure 10.2 Anscore Machine for Testing Autonomic Neuropathy

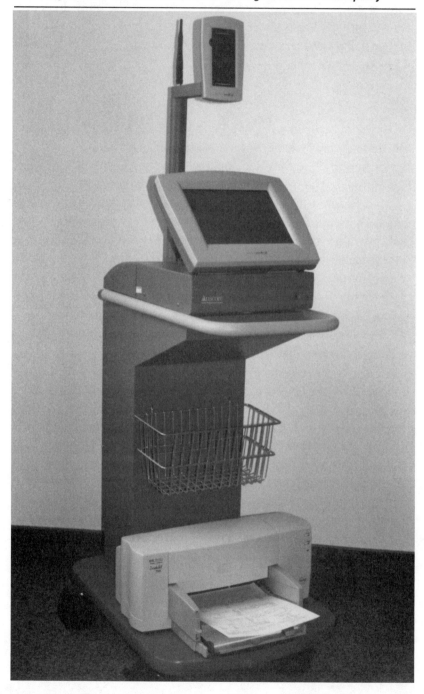

spine or single muscle fibers in various parts of the body. Improvement in either of these is usually seen in three to four months and does not appear to be that closely associated with the normalization of blood-glucose levels.

Radiculopathy

This type of neuropathy begins at the roots of the spinal nerves. Pain or sensory loss may be experienced on any part of the skin surface. The most common place for radiculopathy is the nerves between the ribs. This causes very severe chest pain, especially with breathing. Sometimes it is so severe that the person needs oxygen because of the inability to get a deep breath. There is no treatment except support, but it is non-fatal. It will usually resolve within a week or two, though it can recur in the same nerve or in another nerve later on.

Normalization of blood-glucose levels is the best documented approach to reduce the risk of neurologically related complications. This finding has given added importance to the need to keep blood-glucose values under 150 mg/dl (8.3 mmol) for prevention of problems and for reversal of changes that may have already occurred.

Microangiopathy

Small-blood-vessel disease (microangiopathy) is responsible for many problems related to the kidneys (nephropathy), to the eyes (retinopathy), and to some degree to the muscle of the heart (cardiomyopathy). While heart disease has been associated mainly with macroangiopathy, some microangiopathy also occurs.

Kidney Damage (Nephropathy)

Nephropathy may be associated with infection of the kidneys, ureters, bladder, or urethra. Infection of the urinary tract is common in people with diabetes because of sugar in the urine and/or because urine may be kept in the bladder as a result of neuropathy. If the infection starts in the bladder and either occurs over and over again or goes up the ureters to the kidneys, damage to the kidneys may occur. Any damage to the kidneys will eventually result in decreased kidney function. Diabetic nephropathy (damage of the kidney) is often a result of blood-vessel damage, with scarring of the filtration system of the major part of the kidney. This may be caused by thickening (and thus weakening) of membranes in the blood-vessel walls as a result of elevated blood-glucose levels. Bleeding could occur, and protein could leak from these blood vessels.

Checking for protein in the urine helps in early detection of renal disease (note, however, that protein in the urine is not always due to kidney damage but can also be due to some other stressor, such as infection or intense exercise). Control of hypertension is extremely important, as is prompt treatment of any urinary tract infection.

Diabetic nephropathy is detected by finding protein in the urine. If there is a small amount of protein (called microproteinuria), the condition can be reversed by careful control of blood sugar and blood pressure, especially with drugs called ACE (angiotensin converting enzyme) inhibitors. But if there is a large amount of protein in the urine (called gross proteinuria), then it is too late and the condition can only be slowed, not stopped, and kidney failure is inevitable. Therefore, be sure your doctor follows the American Diabetes Association guidelines and measures microprotein or microalbumin or get an albumin/creatinine ratio at least once a year. It is a simple and inexpensive test and can save your kidneys and possibly your life.

When nonreversible kidney damage has occurred, renal dialysis (cleaning the blood through the use of a machine) or, as a last resort, renal transplant, now offers hope of improved quality and quantity of life. Improved tissue-matching techniques and new immunosuppression drugs (medicine to keep the recipient from rejecting the transplant) have resulted in more successful transplantations.

Retinopathy

Retinopathy may occur in various stages, the earliest of which are more reversible. Stage I involves the formation of a microaneurysm, which is the ballooning of a weak wall of a blood vessel. Microaneurysms may burst and hemorrhage. Exudates, or defined yellow spots, can sometimes be seen on the retina. While these were once thought to be fat or lipid deposits, they have actually been found to be scars from areas of bleeding in the retina. Stage II involves new vessel formation, hemorrhage, and scarring. Once this has occurred, it is not possible to reverse the condition. However, stabilization is possible through laser treatment.

The lens of the eye may also have problems. In the presence of higher glucose levels (blurs vision), the lens can become more translucent than transparent, resulting in the formation of a cataract. The cataract can be easily removed and a new lens transplanted.

If hemorrhage (bleeding) has occurred in the eye, the fluid in the eye may become cloudy. Removal and replacement of this fluid may restore clear vision (vitrectomy). Also, scarlike membranes that have formed on the retina may be surgically removed.

If there is too much pull on the retina, as can occur because of multiple bleeding episodes and subsequent scarring, the retina may pull away from the back wall of the eye. Retinal detachment can be corrected through the scleral buckling procedure, which may include the removal of scar tissue and the refitting of the retina to the back wall of the eye through the placement of fluid in the eyeball to "force" the retina against the inside "wall" of the eye.

Retinopathy need not inevitably cause blindness. When retinopathy is discovered early and treated vigorously, vision can be preserved. Therefore, have a dilated eye exam at least once a year as recommended by the American Diabetes Association guidelines.

Macroangiopathy

Large-blood-vessel disease most often affects the heart, but it may also affect the brain or the extremities. Heart attack, angina (pain), and coronary artery disease are related to damage to large (macroangiopathy) and small (microangiopathy) blood vessels. The blood vessels feeding the heart can become obstructed, resulting in death of part of the heart muscle, causing a heart attack (cardiovascular disease).

You may have heard of the diagnosis called syndrome X. Although the first reporting of this syndrome, by Dr. George Reavens, included only arteriosclerosis, hyperlipidemia, hyperglycemia, obesity, and hypertension as increased risk factors for cardiovascular disease, this syndrome now also includes an increase in insulin release, an increase in insulin resistance, serum uric acid elevation, an increase in smaller, dense VLDL (very low density liproproteins), an increase in low-density lipoproteins, a decrease in high-density lipoproteins, and an increase in plasmino-activator inhibitors. New names for syndrome X are metabolic syndrome, dysmetabolic syndrome, and prediabetes.

Various treatments can help greatly in the prevention of, stabilization of, and/or recovery from these occurrences, especially heart attacks. Coronary dilation, plaque removal, Stent insertion, ballooning, coronary artery bypass graphs (CABG), as well as drugs such as vasodilators, alpha and beta blockers, ACE inhibitors (angiotensin converting enzyme inhibitors), and calcium channel blockers are the currently used tools. These "tools" are accompanied, as needed, with uric acid and cholesterol and triglyceride controlling medications, along with the various methods of controlling hyperglycemia.

Be aware of the fact that large vessel disease with resultant problems such as heart attacks can occur at an early age, especially in females who have diabetes. A young woman with diabetes can have a heart attack at a much earlier age (even in her twenties) than a woman who does not have diabetes. Good control of blood sugar along with proper diet and exercise is the prevention.

Cerebral Vascular Disease (CVD)

A rupture or blockage of a blood vessel could occur in the brain. Part of the brain would thus not receive adequate nourishment, and unconsciousness or paralysis would result (usually an occurrence in the right side of the head affects the left side of the body).

Peripheral Vascular Disease (PVD)

PVD, as the name implies, is observed in the extremities of the body, such as the arms and legs. PVD can be treated with a variety of techniques, including angioplasty, laser treatment, and bypass grafts. The simplest of these is balloon angioplasty, in which a catheter is placed in the artery and fed to the area of blockage. A balloon is then inflated to squeeze the fatty blockage against the vessel wall and open the vessel.

Intermittent claudication (cramping pain on walking due to partial blockage of the blood vessels) is associated with disease affecting the legs. Hardening of the arteries (arteriosclerosis) can involve any large blood vessel. If the blood can't get through, the loss of the affected part of the body is possible. Any pain or decreased blood flow (pain, redness, blackness or blueness) in the lower extremities should immediately be called to the attention of your physician.

General Information

Complications, whether acute, intermediate, or chronic, can usually be prevented or controlled. Much is being done to prevent and overcome these problems. Your participation at any stage of development of such a problem will assist you in achieving better or at least more stable health. It is important that you keep aware of any changes in your body, as well as changes in treatments that might be of help to you.

Over a nine-year period, the Diabetes Control and Complications Trial investigators tested and observed 1,441 people who were divided into study groups. There were two major groups: insulin-dependent people who had no signs of complications of diabetes and an insulin-dependent group who had early signs of diabetes retinopathy. These major groups were then subdivided into groups labeled "Intensive Control" and "Conventional Control" (see Appendix K for definitions). The results of the study, reported during the American Diabetes Association's national meeting in June 1993, were as follows: In the Intensive Control group there was a 76 percent reduction in the risk of having eye disease (retinopathy), a 53 percent reduction in the risk of having kidney disease (nephropathy), a 61 percent reduction in the risk of having nerve disease (neuropathy), and a 35 percent reduction of the risk of developing a high level of bad cholesterol (LDL). The average hemoglobin A1c was 7.2 percent in the Intensive Control group (versus 8.9 percent in the Conventional Control group).

The downside was weight gain and three times the occurrence of severe hypoglycemia. The upside? Intensive control can be achieved, but it requires hard work, a well-motivated person, and a well-trained health care team.

Another study that included a larger number of people over a longer period of time was the United Kingdom Prospective Diabetes Study (UKPDS). This important study was done with people with Type 2 diabetes and involved over 5,000 people over several years. There were many subgroups with different medications, but the results were the same: For every one point drop in the A1c, there was a 25 percent decrease in long-term complications. The same was true for control of blood pressure.

So the lessons learned from these studies and others are:

- Keep your blood pressure in the normal range (less than 130/80).
- Keep your blood sugars in the normal range as much as possible (hemoglobin A1c less than 7 percent).
- Keep your high-density lipoproteins above 45 and your low-density lipoproteins below 100 (lipid profile).

Guidelines to follow include:

- Ask for a hemoglobin A1c test every three to four months (or at least twice a year).
- Have a thorough foot exam once a year (or at each visit if you have lost feeling in your feet).
- Have your urine tested for microalbumin or albumin/creatinine ratio once a year if the test for protein in the urine indicating 200 mg/dl or above protein (gross proteinuria) has not been noted. If there is 200 mg/dl or above, then a twelve- or twenty-four-hour urine test for creatinine clearance (the processing of urine through your kidneys) and total protein is noted (multi-chem needed).
- Ask for a referral to a nephrologist if creatinine is 2.0 or above or if blood pressure is not controllable.
- Have a dilated eye examination once a year starting the first year with a Type 2 diagnosis and after five years of diagnosis with Type 1.

With these and other methods developed for early detection of developing problems, you will have a greater chance of reducing the risk of having the complications too often associated with this disease syndrome.

11

How Do You Adjust to Having Diabetes?

How do you adjust to the diagnosis of diabetes or to being told that you have one or more of the complications of the disease?

Reacting to the Diagnosis

If you have just received the diagnosis of diabetes or if you have just heard of someone else with diabetes who is suffering from a variety of problems, you may be somewhat fearful. You know that having this disease will have a significant impact on your life and on your family's life. As our mentor, Dr. Robert L. Jackson, has stated, "This is a disease that has the potential of helping families to grow." As complicated as the management program may seem, Dr. Jackson feels that it can be fairly simple: eating nutritious foods to meet the needs of growth and activity levels, taking the amount of medication needed to cover the food and activity, and testing to see whether the decisions have been correct.

When you are first diagnosed, it is not helpful to you when others say that at least it's better than having cancer (or some other disease), however true this may be. Even when they say, "You'll become more healthy because you'll learn how to really take care of yourself," it does not help at first. You're too emotionally involved to be ready to learn at this point. Perhaps you'll even find yourself saying some of these things to others about your diagnosis. Your family and friends may feel awkward around you. You can guide them by telling them that they don't need to say anything; they just need to support you. Simply saying "I'm sorry this has happened to you" or giving you a hug can be enough at this time. Talking to another person who has had diabetes or meeting with a support group for a while helps, too. (See Appendix I for help in finding a contact near you through your local diabetes chapter of your state affiliate.)

Seek out support people—those with whom you can talk comfortably and to whom you can display your true feelings and thoughts.

Ask your family to keep junk food out of the house; to not tempt you by offering you sweets; to give you an injection now and then (if you were really ill, their knowing how to do this would come in handy); to learn how to treat an insulin reaction; and, especially, for immediate family members, to attend diabetes education classes with you.

When the emotional edge subsides and you can start asking questions, then go to a source to learn as much as you can.

If you feel that you really haven't adjusted to the diagnosis of diabetes or to having a complication of the disease, consider some other ways of thinking. Consider the ways of healthy living that are part of your control of diabetes. This knowledge could be shared with others. In the case of a complication, consider being grateful that the complication was discovered at an early stage, if true, or that stabilization of the complication is more possible now than it was ten years ago. Consider talking to a counselor, pastor, or psychologist. There may never be an answer that satisfies you, but once you can accept the reality that you have diabetes or a complication, grasp this as a challenge, then get actively involved. As noted earlier, in some situations early diagnosis of a complication and improvement of diabetes control can reverse or slow the progress of the complication.

The Grief Response

You may feel angry or depressed. These emotional responses are common, and it is all right to have—and to recognize—these emotions. People respond in varying ways to news that is not considered pleasant. This response is often termed "the grief response." The grief response includes the emotional responses of denial, anger, bargaining, depression, and acceptance. These may occur in sequence, or some may be experienced at the same time or in a different order. Allow the grief process to occur. Don't try to be superhuman or stoic. Remember that the grief response is natural and that it is okay for your family as well as you to have such feelings.

Denial This is often the initial response to diagnosis. Denial might be expressed as "It's not really true."

Anger This is often expressed as "Why me?" Anger can occur at the same time as denial. The diagnosis might be blamed on a family member, on an accident, on stress at work, or on some other factor.

Bargaining Bargaining involves weighing the odds. Most often, the person denies that choices made today will influence his or her health status later on.

Depression This emotion seems to reappear time and time again, with varying intensity. Depression noted shortly after diagnosis of the disease appears to reach some resolution in six to nine months for children and one to two years for an adult. Reminders of the disease (for example, medical costs, diagnosis of a complication, monitoring blood sugars, and clinic visits) may trigger depressive episodes. The person may even decide not to monitor blood-sugar levels or see the health care professional.

Acceptance This is a time of resolution. Denial is no longer present, and the person asks what she or he needs to do to get on with life. Acceptance signifies the person's readiness to learn.

Let's return to discussing depression. This emotional response is often misunderstood. There are two types of depression: pathological and functional. Pathological depression occurs when a person is no longer able to make rational decisions, talks less or stops talking altogether, or withdraws. Surprisingly, this occurs no more or less often in persons with diabetes than in the nondiabetic population. Functional depression is considered less severe and is usually resolved with education and support.

Defense Mechanisms

Anger, denial, and bargaining may be associated with responses called *defense mechanisms*. The major defense mechanisms are rationalization, regression, reaction formation, repression, withdrawal, and compensation.

Rationalization means saying, for example, that something desired but not obtained was no good, anyway.

Regression, which is more noticeable in adults than in children, means becoming more dependent on other people to cook food, give shots, monitor the disease, make decisions, and so forth. Or a person may regress by not taking appropriate care of himself or herself.

Reaction formation can be described as a person's doing the opposite of what he or she has been told to do. For example, if told to decrease caloric intake, this person responds by "pigging out."

Repression means that a person "forgets" what he or she is supposed to do, either subconsciously or consciously. An example of repression is a person "forgetting" to take insulin.

Withdrawal represents a more acute state of depression. A person may feel that all is hopeless and may therefore do nothing at all.

Compensation, which is a positive defense mechanism, means taking a negative or a handicap and actually making a positive out of it. The person works harder to overcome something that, by some standards, would be considered an obstacle rather than an opportunity. Compensation is one way of reframing, or looking at something (such as a statement or action) in a different light. For example, while having a chronic illness is a definite negative, you could look at how healthy you have become through improved self-care routines. With skill, you can take almost any situation or thought and reframe it in a positive way.

Parents of children who have been diagnosed with diabetes commonly report feelings of guilt: "I somehow gave this to my child." Some parents rebel against this feeling by acting out in ways that make the child feel rejected. Through their actions, such parents are stating, "My child is less than perfect. This child is no longer mine." Parents need to recognize that in our present state of knowledge, there is nothing that can be done to prevent a child from developing diabetes.

Self-Esteem

Your self-esteem involves who you think you are, what strengths you feel you have, and what you feel you have achieved. Your level of self-esteem will have a great deal to do with how you react to having diabetes. If you have low self-esteem you may feel overwhelmed, become too dependent, be afraid of change, and even, through poor choices, be self-destructive. Or you might respond in an opposite manner, being too boastful or ignoring other people's feelings. In either case, you need to improve your level of self-esteem.

Your self-esteem can be assessed by considering your mental, emotional, and physical self. This assists you in developing a realistic image of yourself. Once you accept yourself as you are, you can take pride in the things you have done. Your activities and accomplishments assist you in developing self-confidence—a very important part of self-esteem. Recognize that it is all right to fail, and that you have the courage to learn from failure and go on. You may have felt guilt about failing. Recognize that guilt is a thing of the past. Use it as a learning experience about yourself, without condemning yourself.

You can improve your self-esteem by developing knowledge about your good points. Use these good points to assist you in enhancing your self-confidence. Become a friend to yourself. Know that you are a unique being. Choose to risk allowing yourself to grow.

Family Support

There are a number of things you can do to support yourself and that your family can do to help support you. The first step is to aid your family in recognizing that diabetes is an illness that will not disappear. Get some help for all of you if you or they seem to be dwelling on any part of the grief process. A professional therapist or counselor can support and guide you and your family through the thinking process. Most of all, allow you and your family time.

Adjusting to any disturbing news takes time. You may want to think about going to a diabetes camp, either as a camper or a counselor (see Appendix J for the name of the American Diabetes Association camp closest to you). Encourage your family members to learn as much as they can. Help them to learn the definitions of diabetes-related terms (see Appendix K). Encourage them to attend chapter meetings of the American Diabetes Association. Both you and they can become support persons for others.

Some people say they have never adjusted to having diabetes. Others, however, say that once they and their family reached the point of acceptance, they chose to fight the disease and its potential consequences with all the weapons available to them. One of the most important weapons is family support. Such people choose to feel that they are controlling their diabetes rather than that the disease is controlling them.

12

How Does Stress Affect Diabetes?

Anyone who has diabetes must become aware of anything that encourages the release of glucose into the bloodstream. The result is an elevated blood sugar. This physical response is different in each person, due to individual emotional and physical factors as well as environmental considerations. As already noted, being diagnosed with diabetes is stressful, as is being told that you have a complication of the disease. Having various pressures in life that influence the control of the disease is also stressful. Any event or information could be the "stressor." Any physical response you have to that event or information is called *stress*. When you experience stress, your body usually responds by circulating blood faster. Glucose is "poured" from its storage sites (the liver and muscle sites) into the bloodstream. Your blood pressure increases, as does your pulse rate (except in a frustrated type of stress response, in which your pulse rate may actually slow down). A variety of signs and symptoms may be noted, including dilation of the pupils.

Acute Response

The most frequent, rapid response a person experiences during stress is called the alarm (or acute) response. It is termed "acute" because the adrenaline release occurs within a short time. The brain sends a message to the adrenal gland, telling it to secrete adrenaline. This adrenaline release, which may take from seconds to minutes, occurs when the blood glucose is too low, when the person is scared or excited, or when the body thinks it is at risk. When adrenaline is released, there are many physiological responses. Adrenaline stimulates an increase in heart and pulse rate. It is also indirectly responsible for the cooling effect of the body (perspiration). Blood vessels in the hands and feet narrow. For the person with diabetes, the most common responses experienced with hypoglycemia are due to adrenaline release. This adrenaline release results in weakness, shakiness, and a strong, rapid pulse.

These symptoms stop when the blood-glucose levels rise to normal. When the sugar in the system is already high, the person usually feels the response of high blood sugar rather than the adrenaline released. The major purpose of adrenaline release in a person with diabetes is the subsequent release of glucose into the bloodstream. It is thus both a blessing and a curse: a blessing in raising low blood sugar, and a curse in adding to the problems of diabetes control by rapidly raising the blood sugar above normal (as in the case of brittle diabetes, discussed later in the next section).

Chronic Response

In most cases, the acute response rebalances the body, making the person able to deal with the problem at hand. The chronic (day-to-day) problems associated with having diabetes affect the body somewhat differently. A little cortisol release is helpful; a lot is not. Cortisol is a steroid type of hormone, released from the outside section of the adrenal gland. The body's response to cortisol is to increase blood pressure and to decrease the pulse rate. Other things that happen are a decrease in the number of white blood cells and an increase in the rate that amino acids (protein) change into sugar (glucose). The release of these cortisol types of hormones occurs in minutes to hours.

Other hormones in the body that affect the blood-glucose levels, either directly or indirectly, are glucagon, thyroid-stimulating hormone, and growth hormone. Growth hormone is released even in adults. The result is a greater mobilization of fats for energy, leaving glucose in the bloodstream. All of these counterregulatory hormones wreak havoc on blood-sugar control. Even when no food is eaten, blood-sugar levels can be high at one time and low at others. Some doctors have termed this "brittle diabetes." Others call individuals who experience this "hyper-responders." Whether it has to do with lifestyle or with poor management, the results are the same.

Other Responses

Although there are multiple factors that lead to the physical stress response, it has been found that these factors are not as simple as originally described by the world-renowned father of the stress management field, Dr. Hans Selye. Multiple causes, which vary from person to person, are responsible for the body's physical, mental, and emotional responses. Dr. Selye's General Adaptation Syndrome can be adapted to assist you in understanding why you feel the way you do when your blood sugar is low, and why your body becomes your own enemy when your blood sugar is high.

The first phase is rightly called the *alarm phase*. The feelings you get could be associated with acute happenings such as diabetic ketoacidosis and hypoglycemia. The feelings are most noticeable when you are hypoglycemic. Blood pressure rises, the pulse rate increases, and you feel shaky, nervous, tense, and anxious. Sugar is made available to the body due to an adrenaline release.

The second phase is *resistance*. This is associated with the release of steroid-like hormones. The person has a sense that nothing can be done. If a person diagnosed with diabetes has difficulty adjusting to the disease physically, mentally, and emotionally, self-care may be ignored. The chronic high blood sugars lead to changes in the body cells, which can lead to complications.

The third phase is *exhaustion*. While complications during the other phases are usually reversible, in this phase they are less so. If control is established so that stability is maintained, a little improvement might be noted, but problems are still likely. However, in individual cases in which there have been some eye, kidney, and neurological changes, some women have chosen to become pregnant once these problems have been contained. With teamwork, a positive outcome of a healthy baby and a stable mother has been shown to be possible. Keeping the blood-glucose levels normal throughout the pregnancy can thus enable a woman to have a good pregnancy despite her body's being in the exhaustion phase of stress due to diabetes.

Stress Management

What can you do about stress? There are a number of ways to handle it. Taking responsibility for yourself by becoming your own PARENT is one.

Positive Thinking

Believe it or not, you can increase the release of the hormone endorphin, which leads to increased physical strength, if you think positively. If you consider a person you know to be a negative thinker, you may also recognize how frequently that person is ill. Positive thinking is thus associated not only with physical strength but also with an improved level of health. Positive thinking may include prayer, meditation, affirmations, and humor (don't forget, humor is healing).

Attitude

Your attitude comes from the beliefs you have and thus develops from the inside out. Your attitude affects your diabetes by supporting you to make correct choices. Therefore, a good attitude is very important in self-management. The "A" in PARENT also stands for assertiveness. You must be assertive in many situations for your own health and safety. Learning conflict resolution and negotiation skills will help you to be more assertive.

Relaxation

There are many ways to relax. These may be partial relaxation or complete relaxation. It is interesting that after spending much of our lives conditioning ourselves to respond to stress, most of us actually need training to learn how to relax properly. First, you need to become aware of whether what you are currently doing to relax is really relaxing to you. Check this out by getting an alcohol thermometer. Hold the bulb lightly between the thumb and forefinger until the red-dyed alcohol is stable, indicating the present body temperature of your hands (this is called "peripheral body temperature"). This temperature indicates how relaxed you are. When the temperature of your fingers is in the seventies or low eighties, it usually means that you are more tense (or cold!). When it is either in the nineties or four degrees higher than your previous temperature, you are more relaxed. The more the peripheral blood vessels open (dilate), the more the muscles have relaxed and the more blood flows unobstructed to your fingertips.

After you have noted this temperature, do what you normally do to relax (for example, read, watch TV, walk, or work on a hobby project). After ten or twenty minutes, sit quietly for about a minute with your hands in your lap, then take your peripheral body temperature again. If you have relaxed, this second temperature should be two to four degrees higher than the first temperature, as noted earlier. If the temperature hasn't changed or is lower than the previous temperature, note that the activity you tested, while not necessarily bad, is not an activity to undertake if you want to relax your body.

The training goal of relaxation is to get into a state in which you "get out of your own way." Any process may be used, but all approaches must have one thing in common: They must focus your mind on something other than your problems. Deep breathing, progressive relaxation, autogenic therapy, meditation, imaging, and biofeedback are some of the techniques that can be used. The training process for these techniques takes anywhere from six to ten weeks, with practice periods of ten to twenty minutes, preferably twice a day.

Deep Breathing Two to three deep breaths are taken for immediate release of tension. For deeper relaxation, seven to eight breaths are recommended. This is deep, abdominal breathing, and lightheadedness can occur if you get up too quickly at the end of the breathing practice time.

Progressive Relaxation This is a process of contracting and relaxing the muscles, beginning with the toes and moving up to the face. You learn to sense how the muscles feel by contracting them for ten to twenty seconds and sensing how they feel in that contracted state, then relaxing these same muscles and sensing how they feel in the relaxed state.

Autogenic Therapy In this approach, you imagine that your muscles are very heavy (relaxed). (The same muscle sequence used for progressive relaxation can be followed.) When the muscles surrounding the blood vessels are relaxed, these muscles become warmer due to unobstructed blood flow. This is a physical, or mechanical, response rather than an imagined response. Statements such as "My arms are heavy and warm" assist in this process.

Meditation Traditionally, the focus here is a sight or a sound. For example, a mantra or other specific sound might be repeated over and over again. Dr. Herbert Benson, associate professor of medicine at Harvard, is a leader in the stress management field. Dr. Benson has people focus on the repetition of the word "one" as part of his program involving the "relaxation response." Other people use prayer or a scripture. Still others concentrate on a picture or on a spot on the wall. As relaxation ability improves, the relaxation response can occur within a shorter period of time.

Imagery This technique takes your focus away from your problems. The imaging can take the shape of people, places, or things, or it can involve focusing on bright to calm colors (and back) or bright to calm music (and back). Visualizing an accomplishment, such as climbing a mountain with supportive aid as needed (from family, friends, or spiritual strength), provides a sense of accomplishing a goal and the peace and good feelings that accompany it.

Biofeedback Biofeedback is a technique in which you learn to use information about changes in your body. Relaxation training may be enhanced through biofeedback, such as might be obtained by measuring skin resistance, muscle-energy output, or temperature of the hands or feet. The initial use of biofeedback is just to let you know how you are responding to changes in thought or position. Later on, it aids in training you to become more relaxed by letting you know which types of activities represent your "getting out of your own way" so that your body automatically relaxes. The key is not to try. (Remember what happens when you try to go to sleep? You are more wide awake. Similarly, if you try to relax, you will become more tense.) Instead, allow yourself to become relaxed by focusing your thoughts away from the hectic problems of the day.

Dr. Herbert Benson's program is simple, especially after you've learned to do deep abdominal breathing, and requires only two steps. The first is to repeatedly *say, look,* or *think* about something: a scripture, a poem, a rosary, or a prayer. The second step is to passively handle intrusive thoughts. This means peacefully telling yourself that this is your quiet time and you will think about "whatever" at the end of the session. A session of ten to twenty minutes once or twice per day will result in lower blood pressure, a slower pulse rate, and a more efficient use of oxygen.

Exercise

Exercise not only helps you to feel good about yourself, but, when done on a daily or every-other-day basis, as noted before, can reduce depression, increase the pain threshold, and improve cardiovascular strength. To be effective as a form of stress management, the exercise must be participated in for twenty to thirty minutes daily or every other day. When you are mentally tired, exercise will act as a stimulant. When you want to be more creative and more organized, exercise will stimulate these attributes. Too much exercise, or exercise performed when the body is in a stressed state (that is, with blood-sugar levels of 250 mg/dl [14 mmol] or greater, or during illness), will only lead to a stressed state or aggravate the existing stressed state. Exercising wisely can aid in decreasing the physical stress responses of the body. Be sure that food and/or nutrients are timed and are in the proper amounts to give you the best support. Yoga, tai chi, and qi gong are good exercise options.

Nutrition

Nutrition is perhaps one of the most important antistressors available. Good nutrition is really very subtle in its actions. Just as with diabetes, outwardly you may not be aware of any difference, but inwardly the body is responding differently. As you become more aware of the impact of nutrition on your body, you will notice changes in skin tone, a sense of alertness, less bloating or other intestinal problems, and so forth. For stress management, you need to think not only about how much you eat but also about what you eat, when you eat, and how fast you eat.

As with earlier advice on nutrition, most of the directions for nutrition related to stress management apply to the nondiabetic person as well.

How is nutrition useful as an antistressor? Eating the appropriate amount for the activity or for growth and development is helpful. An overloaded stomach leads to sluggish thinking and sluggish activity. The composition of the food determines the nutritional status of the body. Purposefully planning to replace nutrients that have been used or to take in the right nutrients at the right time leads to better health. Eating at erratic times can throw the body out of balance, not only in terms of the digestive functions but also in terms of the action time of medication taken to control blood-glucose levels. Sweets are empty calories and don't make you feel good. And too much of any one food—whether it is sweets, high fiber, or anything else—can throw your body out of balance and result in some physical effects.

Remembering that the best nutrition is obtained from whole foods, if there are deficits or important health needs in your diet, vitamins (the American Medical Association recommends one multivitamin a day), minerals, or herbs might be useful. Also, caution must be exercised concerning other medications you are taking and if you have kidney (nephropathy) or liver problems. Learn before you try. Talk with a knowledgeable person. As much as possible, add only one megavitamin, mineral, or herb at a time to be sure they fit with your body's present functioning.

Touch

There are a variety of definitions for the term *touch*. If you reach out to others, you in turn feel the effect in yourself. Touch also relates to therapeutic massage—that is, the loosening of muscles through touch so that you achieve a relaxed state both physically and mentally. Massage can give relief to tense and stiff muscles, and it can increase joint flexibility and range of motion. It aids in reducing blood pressure. It can assist in improving the capacity for clear thinking, and it gives a feeling of well-being.

Another form of "touch" is therapeutic touch. Therapeutic touch was first taught by Dora Kuntz and Dr. Delores Krieger (Nurse Healers Professional Association, 801-273-3339). In a sense, it involves very little actual physical touch but is a way to determine, restore, and smooth the energy fields of the body.

Healing touch is a process that includes a variety of techniques. Janet Mentgen, the founder, first taught this process (International Healing Touch Association, 323-989-7982).

You could learn to do one or more of these techniques to help yourself or to aid another person or to teach another person to do it for you when you are in some discomfort or just need to relax. The bibliography at the end of this book includes books that can help you to understand and learn more about these therapies.

Then there is the exhilarating touch of giving or receiving a hug. A hug increases the heart rate and circulation and aids in an all-around feeling of being "okay." June Biermann and Barbara Toohey prescribe four hugs a day. Others have stated that we all need four hugs a day for survival, eight hugs for maintenance, and twelve hugs for growth!

Stress management involves taking responsibility for yourself—for your thoughts and your actions. It means that you may become more mature, that you are able to take the "good news" of self-care and turn it into a level of self-management that leads to a healthier mind and body.

As you learn how to include stress management in your own life and how to relax, you may find that your blood-sugar levels are getting lower and more stable. Keep in touch with your health professional(s), since less medication may be needed.

13

How Can You Help Your Health Care Team Help You?

The total management package for people with diabetes requires a team effort. Like any management package, diabetes management requires all parts to function: physical, mental, emotional, and spiritual. Most of all, it requires you to follow directions, think through your program, and have input into that program. Nothing can happen without interaction between you and your physician (and other health team members). Some of the additional team members are the nurse in the hospital or clinic, the nurse educator (preferably a certified diabetes educator), the dietitian, the pharmacist, the counselor or psychologist, the social worker, the podiatrist, and the exercise specialist. You should find out if the nurse, dietitian, and/or pharmacist are recognized as advanced diabetes practitioners.

Program Management

You are the key person in your program development. The doctors and nurses in the hospital or clinic see that you get the right medication at the right time and that you are monitoring yourself to the best of your ability. The nurse educator works closely with the physician and other health professionals to coordinate resources in the hospital or office and to assist you in carrying out your program at home. The dietitian makes sure that you know what your food choices are and why and when you should eat certain foods. The counselor or psychologist (or psychiatrist, if medication, psychoanalysis, or neuropsychiatric assistance is needed) is on the team to assist you in your adjustment to having a chronic illness and in thinking through the impact it will have not only on your life but also on the lives of your family and friends. The social worker's job is to assist you in the financial realm and in developing or mobilizing community support. This person might also be involved in some counseling, especially for rehabilitation services, if needed. The podiatrist is included to be sure that one of the most vulnerable areas of your body—your feet—are kept in good condition. The exercise specialist helps you to develop your individual exercise prescription, which includes the type of exercise and its frequency, timing, and intensity.

Other key specialists, if they are needed, might include a cardiologist (heart), a nephrologist (kidneys), a neurologist (nerves), an ophthalmologist or retinologist (eyes), a gastroenterologist (stomach, intestines), and an orthopedist (bones).

All care must, of course, be kept in balance. To do this, you must test your blood sugar regularly and monitor your food intake, your activity, and your medicine. You must take note of the way you feel and of whether you have had a reaction. You also need to be aware of any other factors that can help you to personalize your program or that can impact your program, such as the taking of herbs, vitamins, or minerals. (Hopefully your health care professional will be knowledgeable enough to add some of these to your program if they would really help.)

The information must be correct and complete. Accurate input from you, even though it may seem embarrassing at times to give this, will allow your physician and other health professionals to design the most useful and safe program to meet your needs.

Record Keeping

To help the health team help you, you should be sure that your records are as accurate and complete as possible (see Table 13.1). These records also act as a teaching tool for you: Accurately obtained and kept, such data can give you assurance concerning how food and insulin or other diabetes medication result in changes in your blood-glucose levels.

Table 13.1 Monitoring Record

Name _____ Phone _____

Address _____

Date	Time	Time	Time	Time	Time	Comments
Blood sugar						
Ketone						

Date	Time	Time	Time	Time	Time	Comments
Blood sugar						
Ketone						

Sample

Date	Time	Time	Time	Time	Time	Comments
3/3/03	7:00 A.M.	10:00 A.M.	2:30 A.M.	6:30 A.M.	3:00 A.M.	
Blood sugar	110	94	290	110	Not done	
Ketone			Neg.			

To best accomplish the feat of record keeping, look to some of the various companies that offer free blood-glucose monitoring booklets or develop your own on paper or on a computer. Be sure to have your name and some identifying information in the booklet, such as an address or phone number. This information will help in the return of this valuable data should it become lost.

The next two important items are dates and times. There should be places to record variations in information about foods, times, type of low-blood-glucose response, and so on. In recording, the columns should be set up so that you could see a pattern, if one exists. For example, you might find that at 11:45 A.M. every day you have an insulin reaction or that you have a blood-sugar level greater than 200 at 3:00 every afternoon. This would give you guidance as to the need for a change in food or insulin or an oral hypoglycemia agent prior to that time. Use monitors that also have the capacity to display potential patterns of blood sugars and other useful information (having another monitor that quickly gives a blood-sugar reading might be most useful when hypoglycemic).

In some programs you will be given guidance, within set limits, to alter your food, medication, or activity prior to the time a pattern occurs. If you saw that each day, at about the same time, you were having a higher blood sugar (e.g., 204 mg/dl [11 mmol]), you would learn to increase insulin, decrease food, or increase activity prior to the time of day the elevated sugar had been noted. The greater the number of tests done, the greater the ability of the physician to help you. It has been shown that the more one conducts tests and then contacts the health professionals or makes educated changes, the more normal the blood-glucose levels are.

In any case, be sure to have at least three days of what we'll call "profiles." A "profile" means performing a minimum of four blood-glucose tests per day at the predetermined times (for example, fasting and two hours after each meal, or premeal and bedtime). If you are on the "graduate level" of self-management, such information will help you to learn how much insulin by units "covers" a certain amount of calories or carbohydrates in relation to an activity planned for later in the day. These records, along with other information such as the glycosylated hemoglobin test and glycosylated protein or fructosamine levels, will aid in the decision-making process to determine whether to change or maintain your present program.

It is extremely import to record (once things are under control), and promptly report the occurrence of any severe insulin reactions. Most of the time, you will be able to recognize why a severe reaction has occurred. If you are not able to determine why a severe reaction occurred, a change in management is needed right away.

If a change has occurred in your lifestyle, if you plan to travel (especially for the first time after diagnosis), or if you are experiencing a lot of stress and you find that, even though you have followed through with your program, the desired glycemic response is not occurring most of the time, you need to report to your management team so that they can assist you in making changes in your program. Tell them the problem, and, as needed, give them the last two to three days of blood-sugar readings and urine ketone results if a blood-sugar reading has been greater than 250 mg/dl (13.8 mmol). Also tell them of any changes in your food intake or activity.

Case Report

One woman, who had attended a diabetes education program and learned the importance of record keeping and self-management choices, went to her clinic appointment with her well-kept record booklet. Her physician looked briefly at the booklet and then told her that she didn't need to bring in so much information. As the woman was walking out of the office, she saw the physician drop her booklet into the wastebasket. She was so shocked that she turned around, picked up the record booklet, left the office, and promptly changed physicians. The physician probably did not know how to interpret the data, so the woman was wise to find a physician who could interpret the data and support her in achieving optimal blood-glucose level control.

One Final Word

No matter how insignificant a particular piece of information may seem to you, it may be most helpful in assisting your diabetes team to help you. To keep your diabetes from being an obstacle in your life, at a minimum, you need to do three things: (1) monitor; (2) record; and (3) report.

14

How Can You Help Your Family and Friends Help You?

Your diagnosis of diabetes mellitus affects not only you but your family and friends as well. This "ripple effect" is due to the time and energy you need to take good care of yourself. While you need support from your family and friends, in time they will need to be supported, too. It goes both ways. With support going each way, the necessary physical and emotional adjustments can become a part of everyday activity, planning, and thought.

Increasing Their Understanding

Be sure a family member or friend goes with you when you attend diabetes education classes. (As mentioned earlier in this book, when you are questioning what was said, two heads are better than one.) In this way, the other person will also have the opportunity to learn what to expect, what is involved, how to treat an insulin reaction, and how to prevent subconscious sabotage of your program.

This last item is perhaps one of the most important. That "one little bite won't hurt you" comment can lead to more bites of food than are desirable for you. If friends or family do either too much for you (smothering you) or too little (ignoring you and your disease), you may feel upset. Both situations are unhealthy for you, mentally and emotionally.

You need to be educated to the point at which you become independent in your own self-care. If everything is done for you—your shots, blood-glucose tests, meals, and so forth—then you feel like less of a person. You become more dependent on the other person, and you stop growing. On the other hand, if a family member refuses to discuss your disease and your feelings, shuns your company, or refuses to help you with shots or a blood-sugar test when you are very ill, you will likely feel rejected.

In a healthy, balanced situation, friends and family members support you in self-management. They are willing to give you an injection or blood-glucose test if necessary and to purchase your supplies when you are ill. Hopefully, you can also share some of your feelings with them without their scolding you or getting upset.

Gaining Their Support

You can help your family in many ways, some of which may be quite subtle. One way is to see that your family receives diabetes education. This gives them some understanding of how they can be of assistance. It also gives them a recognition that they have emotional responses to your disease, too, along with guidance for handling these emotions.

Offering to let family members give you a shot or do a blood-sugar test gives them practice in case you really need their assistance at a future time. It also indicates that you trust them enough to allow them to do these procedures. Some people may have real fears about giving an injection. Encourage them to recognize that insulin is a lifesaving medicine. Indirectly, oral agents are lifesaving also.

If someone is still unable to participate in your care, recognize that you may feel some sense of rejection. Try to assess the situation from the other person's standpoint. On the other hand, if you refuse to let a family member or friend give you a shot or do a blood test, do so with some explanation of your fears. If this is not done, the other person may experience a sense of rejection. Your family members and friends need to feel that they are accepted and/or that they are a part of your care.

Family meetings can be most helpful. This is a specified weekly period of time (usually from thirty to forty-five minutes) when family members can meet to exchange ideas, discuss feelings, and work on plans. If children are involved, they should be encouraged to take leadership roles. The meetings also help siblings to understand one another (which is especially helpful if it is a child who has diabetes) and to understand themselves. Sibling rivalry is increased if a sibling doesn't know why the child with diabetes is receiving so much attention.

Try to be as realistically independent as you can about the care of your disease. As soon as you are able to do so, give yourself the majority of your injections, and do most of your blood-glucose tests. Learn your meal plan so that you can make appropriate choices from the food that is served. (Education helps the family to cook more nutritious food if you are not involved in the grocery shopping and cooking.) If you are visiting friends and are offered a food you'd rather not have, you can simply say, "Sorry, but that food does mean things to my blood sugar," or with humor, "My doctor (or nurse, dietitian, or pharmacists) would slap my hands if I even aimed a fork in that direction."

Humor is most helpful in your adjustment and in the adjustment of family and friends. When you are able to joke about yourself, others will feel more comfortable in your presence. If you were to walk into a house and state solemnly, "I have diabetes," chances are that your hosts would be walking on eggshells. Your attitude plays a large part in the attitude of others toward you and toward your diabetes. A joking comment in the right place at the right time can make everyone feel more at ease.

Grieving

You, your family, and your close friends will all experience some grief at the time you are first diagnosed or if any complication is diagnosed. Grieving is a normal part of any feeling of loss. Just as it is for you, it is normal for your family and friends to grieve. Just as you might experience disbelief and denial, so might they. When the reality hits that your diagnosis means a change in schedules and meals and makes it necessary to learn new information, family and friends may respond by not saying anything or by nagging you, walking away from you, or keeping too close. Education and counseling will be useful to them, as perhaps you found such support helpful. They don't need to say anything; they just need to listen.

Complementary and Alternative Choices

Well-meaning relatives and friends may encourage you to try this or question whether you have tried that. Some of these suggestions might be good ones and others might be harmful to your health. More scientific research is being done on many practices, from the use of herbs, vitamins, and minerals to the use of massage, acupuncture, and tai chi. Since a whole book could be written on the subject of alternative and complementary choices (and has been; see the Bibliography), learn what is available. Look it up on the Internet or in your library or bookstore, or better yet contact your health care provider or certified practioner and study this together. Remember, not all you read on the Internet is suitable for a person with diabetes.

If the choice is to use something considered complementary (along with exercise or relaxation training, for example) or alternative (in place of what you are now doing), your special needs should influence your choices. If you have any diabetes complications, especially those that include your liver or kidneys, know that your body may not be able to readily handle the waste products from vitamins, minerals, or herbs. Also note that if you are on other medications, they might interact with some herbs and cause you more harm than help.

The American Diabetes Association recognizes the concerns people have in trying unproven therapies. They developed a position paper, found in the first supplement of each year ("Clinical Practice Guidelines") in the journal *Diabetes Care*. This position paper includes the classification for unproven therapies as "clearly effective, somewhat/sometimes effective or effective for certain categories of patients, unknown/unproven but possibly promising, or clearly ineffective." They came to this specific classification by evaluating the practice (or modality) of use by noting the number and quality of studies performed and by evaluating the potential to help or harm patients.

When considering a complementary or alternative product, check to see if the product is approved by the Food and Drug Administration, whether the modality has been supported by two or more peer-reviewed, scientific publications, or if it is endorsed by an association or a relevant health-related specialty organization.

And remember, *natural* does not always mean *safe*.

15

What Is Being Done to Conquer Diabetes and Improve Its Management?

Research brings hope to all those who have diabetes mellitus and to their families. If no research were being conducted, one would have the sense that no one cared, that no one felt that there was any hope. Hope is the lifeblood of the person with diabetes. Whether it is today or tomorrow, new findings will improve the life of anyone who has diabetes.

Transplants

You have diabetes, and you want it cured. Today, ideas seem to be focused on the use of either a pancreatic or associated transplant, or the implantation of an artificial pancreas.

Transplantation of cells or body parts from one person to another (for example, beta cells; islets of Langerhans, which contain the beta cells; or partial or complete pancreas) has been attempted over the last fifteen years. Drugs that suppress the rejection system of the body (immunosuppression) must be taken once the transplant is in place in order to prevent rejection of the transplant by the body, which recognizes that what has been transplanted is not its own.

Though there has been a lot of progress in the development of anti-rejection drugs in the last few years, they are still very toxic. New drugs have made rejection much less common and transplant much more effective and durable, but the side effects have remained. Since the purpose of the drugs is to prevent the immune system from rejecting the transplanted organ, they must suppress the immune system. This means, at best, the entire or most of the immune system cannot perform its function, which is to kill invading germs and viruses and cancer cells.

Thus, the immunosuppressed person is more susceptible to infection and cancer. In effect, immunosuppression gives the patient a medically induced state of immune deficiency similar to AIDS. True, stopping the medicine, unlike real AIDS, can reverse the immune deficiency state, but then the tissue or organ would be rejected. Because of this serious problem, most of us are not ready to recommend transplant on a very wide scale until there is a better answer to rejection. When a kidney is needed, there is no reason not to go ahead with a transplant if one is available, but to recommend wide-spread transplant in otherwise healthy people is not practical at this time.

The most recent innovation in islet cell transplantation is the Edmonton Protocol. In 2000, researchers in Edmonton, Alberta, published data on eight patients with whom they had used different immunosuppressant drugs (i.e. dropped steroids) and had much better success. With the old protocols using prednisone (a steroid), the graft usually survived less than eight months. With the new protocol without prednisone and a mixture of three relatively new immunosuppressants in low dose, they had a 100 percent survival rate for up to two years. Since then, though success is no longer 100 percent, they have had some grafts survive up to three years and have certainly had much better success than any previous transplant attempts. Several U.S. centers are now using the Edmonton Protocol, and we will watch carefully for their success.

This protocol, while promising and an important step along the road, is still not the final answer. Immunosuppression is still needed and supply of pancreases is a problem. The protocol requires two or sometimes three pancreases for each transplant.

"Pure" beta cells (that is, those that have no attachment to other tissues) have been found to have the least rejection possibilities, but it is impossible at present to completely purify the cells. Thus this immunosuppressant-free form of islet cell transplantation remains elusive.

If a person is given just a part of the pancreas of a living person, the results are similar to the transplant of a kidney or heart. A major surgical procedure is required for both the recipient and the donor, and immunosuppression is needed in the recipient. Whole or partial pancreatic transplants are currently being performed in several centers around the world. Although this procedure has improved the diabetes status of recipients, both rejection and infection are problems.

Dr. David Sutherland, a world-renowned transplant surgeon, has stated that the most effective and long-lasting transplants are those in which the kidney and the pancreas are transplanted at the same time. In over 700 transplants performed since 1978, there has been an 85 percent success rate for simultaneous transplants but only a 75 percent success rate for the transplant of the pancreas alone. (No increase is needed in the immunosuppressant drugs when two organs are transplanted instead of just one.)

The future of transplants may be the use of coated islet cells, or hybrids. With this technology, the islet cells are coated with a semipermeable membrane to protect them from the immune system. Islet cells are purified as much as possible and then covered with an artificial substance that is compatible with body tissue. This substance contains very tiny holes that allow nutrients to enter and wastes and insulin to leave the cells and enter into the circulation. These holes are too small to allow the immune cells or antibodies to enter, thus protecting the islets from rejection. The islets are usually placed in a coating called an alginate made from seaweed and shaped into needle-shaped tubes. The tubes can be inserted under the skin in the abdomen or elsewhere. Another technique for coating cells is to put the cells inside tiny spheres of the membrane material. These spheres can then be transplanted into the abdomen, the spleen, or injected through a vein into the liver. This latter organ is the best place for the spheres and allows insulin to enter the liver before going out in the system, which is the way it happens in nondiabetic people.

In a hybrid system being developed in Canada, the cells are grown on the outside of tiny tubules made of the membranes. These tubules are connected to an artery and a vein to provide circulation. The whole system is enclosed in a plastic box that protects the cells and is then implanted in the abdomen. Much research needs to be done in this area. We are not as yet sure we have the right coating agents, the right number of cells to transplant, and the right location for the cells. Research in islet cell transplantation continues in many locations, but funding is inadequate and restrictions are great.

Availability of pancreases is also a problem, whether for transplant of a whole or partial pancreas, for beta cells, or for islet cells for research. Pancreases for transplant, whether whole, partial, or cells, must come from the same source as other organs (i.e., accident fatalaties). If every pancreas from this source could be harvested, we would still have only enough to transplant fewer than 5,000 persons per year, too few to even make a dent in the number (2,500 per day in the United States) of persons newly diagnosed with diabetes each year. A severe rationing system would then be needed. Such a system would be unfair and not practical.

Growing cells in tissue culture may someday solve the supply problem. Pancreas cells can be cloned or made from stem cells or grown from pancreatic ducts if the proper chemicals are added. Research in this area in several centers, including the Joslin clinic in Boston, Massachusetts, has been promising.

In the meantime, we need to learn to transplant cells from animals. For people with diabetes, pig pancreases is the logical answer since pig insulin is nearly identical to human insulin, and we have used it for years. Before we can consider using animal cells instead of human cells, however, we must solve several problems. The first problem is the cell coating problem to prevent rejection, and the second is the problem of pig viruses. Pigs carry several viruses that are not harmful to pigs but may be harmful to humans, and a way must be found to identify and eliminate these viruses from the cells before transplantation can occur. Because of the potential virus problem, there is an international moratorium on the use of pig tissue for transplantation until much more is known. We have come a long way and have a long way to go, yet transplantation remains a promising area of research and a bright hope for the future.

Artificial Pancreas Transplants

The artificial pancreas is called a "closed-loop" system because it is self-regulating—that is, it contains all the elements of a real beta cell and can regulate itself in controlling the blood-glucose level. Such a system would consist of a sensor to find the current blood-glucose level, a computer or brain to run the system, a pump to inject the insulin, a reservoir to contain the insulin, and a power source to run the system. Ideally, the system would contain a reservoir of glucose or glucagon to counter low blood sugar. With space-age technology and the miniaturization of computer chips, such a system is becoming more and more possible. The biggest obstacle is finding a glucose sensor that, when placed inside the body, would indicate the blood-sugar level and send a message for the need of insulin, glucose, or glucagon. To date, all the materials tried for an internal sensor are good for only a few days; after that they either run out of chemicals to measure the glucose level or become walled off within the body (covered with fibrous, fatty tissue). The walled-off sensor does not sense the true glucose level and thus does not give accurate information. Several devices to measure the glucose levels in the subcutaneous tissue are currently in use or in development. These devices do not measure blood sugar but rather measure the sugar in the tissue juice just under the skin. They cannot as yet be connected to the pump and are being used as continuous glucose sensors to determine defects in blood-sugar control rather that to control a pump. Recent experiments in France and England have tested a closed-loop pump in two patients, but much work remains to be done.

Once the above obstacles are overcome, the next obstacle will be installing a "fail-safe" system or component to counter any malfunction. This could be a section of the closed-loop system in which glucagon might be injected. The glucagon release, at a preset blood-glucose level, would aid in raising the blood sugar. The main part of a closed-loop system, the pump, is being studied in human subjects. It is about the size of a hockey puck, and it contains a reservoir for concentrated insulin. An internal computer, programmed by an external computer through radio-transmitted signals, directs the release of minute amounts of insulin. The amount of insulin to be released is signaled by the results of the finger-stick blood-sugar test. This device is not a closed-loop system since it has no sensor, but it may someday be connected to a sensor similar to the one described above to create a true closed-loop, self-controlled device.

Research on implantable sensors is progressing well. Several systems have been developed and are in clinical use. These are very tiny needles implanted under the skin. Chemicals in the tip of the needle react with the glucose in the tissue and generate an electrical signal. The process is similar to the process used in most glucose meters. The electrical signal can then be telemetered or wired to a pager or (someday) to a wristwatch-size receiver that can interpret the signal as a glucose value that would then be displayed on the watch.

An alternate system being developed uses a tiny laser beam to drill a microscopic hole in the skin through which a tiny drop of tissue fluid is drawn. The device can then measure the glucose in the fluid in a manner similar to the previously described device. The developers of this device hope to combine in the same wristwatch-size receiver a mechanism to infuse insulin through the skin using a process called *reverse iontophoresis*. This process uses an electrical current to make insulin pass through the skin without a needle stick.

A similar device, called the GlucoWatch, was approved by the Food and Drug Administration and became commercially available in the United States in the summer of 2002. This device measures glucose levels but does not infuse insulin. The GlucoWatch sends an electrical impulse into the skin that causes the skin to leak some tissue fluid. This fluid, which contains levels of glucose similar to that in the blood, is absorbed by a pad, and the glucose level is read by the electrons inside the meter and displayed on a screen. This device is slightly smaller than a pager and is strapped to the arm. While this device gives frequent readouts of the glucose level, we cannot get away from the finger-stick test for blood-sugar levels that must still be done twice a day. The pad on the device must be changed twice a day and each time it is changed a blood-glucose reading must be made to recalibrate the device. Thus two pads and two strips must be used each day, making the device fairly expensive to operate.

New Treatments

Insulins today are more refined and much purer than they were in the past. We are now able to make biogenetic human insulin (growing other cells, such as yeast or certain bacterial cells, and genetically engineering them to make human insulin). However, pure human insulin is shorter acting than less pure pork or beef insulin, so more injections a day are required to provide optimal twenty-four-hour control. New insulins called "designer" insulins have been and are being developed. Humalog (lispro) insulin became available in August 1996 and is currently used in a variety of insulin regimens. It is made by switching the proline and lysine amino acids. In 2001, Aventis company released a long-acting insulin (Lantus or glargine insulin), made by substituting glysine for aspartic acid on the first, or alpha, chain and adding two arginines on the beta chain. Novolog insulin (aspart) became available in 2002. It is made by substituting aspartic acid for proline.

These insulins allow much greater flexibility in designing a regimen specific to each individual's needs. Humalog (lispro) or Novolog (aspart) insulin can be used alone or mixed with NPH. They may also be mixed with lente, ultralente, or regular in almost any combination, but must be administered immediately. We most commonly use it for three- or four-dose insulin schedules (some of which were noted previously in the chapter on medications) as follows: (1) Humalog or Novolog before each meal and NPH or lente at bedtime; (2) Humalog and NPH for breakfast, Humalog or Novolog for lunch and supper, and NPH or lente at bedtime; (3) Humalog or Novolog and NPH at breakfast, Humalog at supper, and NPH or lente at bedtime and (4) Humalog or Novolog at meals and ultralente or Lantus once or twice a day. In addition, we sometimes combine regular with one of the Humalog or Novolog doses such as the supper dose. We have used other schedules as well, such as NPH at noon when breakfast and lunch are close together and lunch and supper are too far apart for the Humalog or Novolog to cover. In brief, Humalog and Novolog are versatile insulins that can be used in combinations to tailor the diabetes treatment to individuals and their needs rather than make them change their lifestyle to fit the insulin.

Lantus, or glargine, insulin is unique in that it has a twenty-four, hour duration of action with essentially no peak. It obtains its longer action from the change in amino acids, as noted earlier. Consequently, this insulin has a total of fifty-three amino acids instead of fifty-one resulting in slower absorption when injected into the body.

This flat twenty-four-hour action more closely mimics the action of the pancreas in producing a continuous flow of a small amount of insulin all day and all night, a process called basal insulin secretion. When this drug is combined with a dose of Humalog or Novolog insulin at each meal, a regimen almost totally mimicking nature can be created. Such a combination adjusted for food intake and activity can provide a physiologic and yet flexible program that results in less fluctuation of blood sugar and much less hypoglycemia. Insulin therapy needs to be much easier and more flexible in order to better tailor the treatment to each individual's needs.

Monitoring Devices

Bloodless meters that measure blood glucose without pricking the finger are an ultimate dream. At Kansas State University, a technology was developed for the food industry using a laser beam to measure the sugar content of fruit and other foods without breaking the skin of the food. Unfortunately, this technology is more difficult to use on humans. Skin thickness varies from person to person, and temperature varies the accuracy. This technology, dubbed "The Dream Beam," is still possible, but it will be some time before it is cheap enough or accurate enough to be of practical use. Look for SugarTrac sometime in 2004.

Alternate site testing in the arm, leg, or earlobe is a reality. Several devices are available and are described in the chapter on glucose-monitoring devices. Recent research indicates that there seems to be a lag time from the blood-sugar readings from arm to finger. The recommendation is if low blood sugar or hypoglycemia is suspected, do a finger-stick rather than test an arm or other part of the body.

Insulin Administration

New ways of administering insulin are now available or under study. Injectors, jet-injectors, and so forth have been improved recently and are becoming cheaper. Disposable syringes with smaller needles that are silicon coated for easier and more painless entry are now available and make giving insulin essentially painless if given by the right technique. Nonetheless, many people dream of another way to give insulin. Four ways being tried are by the nasal route, by inhalation into the lungs, a spray in the mouth, and through the skin. The nasal route has been tried for some time, especially in Europe, but has many limitations such as irritation of the nasal membranes, swelling, stuffy nose, and compromised availability when the person has a cold or allergy. Insulin given through the skin is still an idea without much research to support it. Insulin is too large a molecule to get through the skin easily and may not be practical until new methodologies are available, but it still remains a possibility. Several companies are working on skin patch systems that will open the skin cells, thus allowing the insulin to pass through. None of these systems is in large-scale testing yet, so this technology, while promising, is still some time away. A recent finding in Australia showed that the insulin molecule could be made smaller by passing it through a fluid known as a superconductor (at very low temperatures). This nano-molecule may be able to pass through the skin.

Inhaled insulin is currently under testing on humans. The insulin is inhaled like asthma medications using a similar inhaler. The insulin is a powder or aerosol that is inhaled into the lungs, which are endowed with many blood vessels that can absorb the insulin. The method works, but the proper dose schedule and long-term effects are not known. Only short-acting insulin can be given this way, so one or two shots a day of intermediate or long-acting insulin would still have to be given. There is also an aerosol preparation under test that can be sprayed into the mucous membranes of the mouth and be absorbed. The current estimate is that the tests will be completed in 2003 or 2004.

Therapy for Type 2 Diabetes

Some exciting new therapies have been developed for Type 2 diabetes. New oral hypoglycemic agents are being tested, as are combinations of different oral agents and of oral agents and insulin. New dietary treatment is being developed for weight loss and blood-sugar control. There are new findings about the way insulin works and why the body's system goes wrong. Scientists are currently making good progress in learning about Type 2 diabetes, and we are very optimistic about the future. Metformin, acarbose, miglitol, the meglitinide drugs and the glitazone drugs are the recent results of this research. Other new drugs will soon be available. There are at least 122 new drugs in the research pipeline. Eight new drugs (including drug combinations) have come into clinical use since the last edition of this book, so progress is rapid and promises a better life for all persons with diabetes in the next few months and years. Look for new and better ways to treat your disease in the near future.

If you have an idea for a new diabetes treatment, mention it to your family physician. If it seems feasible in any way, contact your diabetes association for the name of a researcher in your area. Write up your idea. If you have difficulty writing, describe it into a tape recorder or have a face-to-face discussion. Get your idea to that researcher. Don't be afraid of being turned down. Perhaps your idea has already been tried. But again, perhaps no one has tried what you have thought up in exactly the same way. If you have the resources, find out ahead of time whether your idea has been tried before. If not, most researchers who know about diabetes will know whether your idea is new or old.

Education for you and for professionals helps to develop new ideas. The American Diabetes Association has developed a set of medical standards to guide health professionals in diabetes management. As they learn about these standards, they may question them or determine that they would be best carried out another way. In other words, the health professionals will stimulate thinking in regard to what is being done, aid in upgrading what is done, and stimulate ideas for doing things better.

The effort to do things better means that there are people who care, and that change is possible for the person who has the disease. Is it best to learn what causes diabetes, how best to manage it, or how to cure it? For those who have the disease, the cure is the focus; for those with a strong family history of diabetes, prevention is the focus. For ongoing care, ways to treat diabetes are the center of attention. Scientists therefore approach diabetes from all of these angles.

Finding the Cause

If diabetes could be prevented, then there would be no need for special machines or surgical procedures. Finding the cause would pave the way for prevention of diabetes and is thus extremely important.

The diabetes syndrome, in most of its forms, is basically genetic, or inherited. As noted before, however, it may have many other causes (e.g., it may result from surgery, certain medications, or other stressful diseases). Type 2 diabetes is an inherited disease, but the gene of inheritance, and even the chromosomes that carry it, have not been positively identified. Some genes and chromosomes have been identified, but there are probably many genes involved in different forms of Type 2 diabetes. Work to identify them continues, since knowing the cause is the first step to finding a prevention or a cure.

The gene, or genes, for Type 1 diabetes are closer to being identified. Type 1 diabetes, which is associated with the immune system (immunology), is a syndrome of diseases rather than one disease. Immunology is closely associated with inherited traits (genetics). People diagnosed with diabetes are often found to have a family history of the disease. Genetic markers are now being revealed, and it someday may be possible for people to take a blood test that will show whether they are predisposed to get one of the diseases of this syndrome. Perhaps some future research will lead to the ability to make changes in the genes by gene splicing or insertion of new genes, so that a person could avoid both developing the disease and passing it on.

Prevention of diabetes, especially Type 1 diabetes, is a highly desirable goal. A study called the Diabetes Prevention Trial (DPT) is currently under way for this purpose. In DPT-1, first-degree relatives (parents, children, and siblings of persons with Type 1 diabetes) were screened by a blood test that measured antibodies to the pancreas. If these were positive, further testing was carried out to determine how much damage had been done to the beta cells of the pancreas. If these latter tests met certain criteria, the person was randomized to either insulin treatment or "oral" insulin treatment or no treatment. In the treatment group, insulin was given by injection in low doses to see if full-blown diabetes could be prevented. Unfortunately, this phase of the study did not prove to be successful and was discontinued in June 2001. The second part of the study (DPT-2) still continues, although it is not adding any new subjects to the study population.

In DPT-2, first-degree and second-degree relatives (aunts, uncles, cousins, and grandparents) were screened with the blood test and, if positive, were randomized to either an oral form of insulin or a placebo. The purpose of the oral insulin in both groups is not to treat diabetes but to somehow interfere with the immune system and prevent diabetes in those susceptible. DPT-2 and other therapies for the prevention of Type I diabetes, through sponsorship by the National Institutes of Health and by the network of scientists and centers, continues on, especially with the population identified through the DPT-1 study.

Research is progressing rapidly in determining the relationship of the immune system to Type 1 diabetes and developing chemicals to stimulate or suppress the immune system. Although this work is still in its early stages, we are very hopeful that a way to prevent Type 1 diabetes will be found in the not too distant future. We strongly hope that this is the last generation of children who will develop Type 1 diabetes.

There was also a nationwide study on the prevention of Type 2 diabetes. This study was designed to see if Type 2 diabetes is preventable. Known as DPP (Diabetes Prevention Program), it was a study of people who were likely to develop Type 2 diabetes based on screening criteria, such as women with a history of gestational diabetes; people who were obese, had a strong family history of diabetes, and were in certain high-risk ethnic groups; and similar criteria. These individuals were divided into several groups, such as support groups using diet and exercise only, groups taking metformin, and a control group taking no drugs and following no special program. The people were to be followed for five years to see if the incidence of developing full-blown diabetes is different with different forms of prevention. The study was stopped after four years (in spring 2002) because of the remarkable results. Compared to the control group who had no lifestyle changes and took a placebo pill, the lifestyle change (diet and exercise) group had a 60 percent reduction in progression to diabetes. The metformin group had a 30 percent reduction. Their results were especially striking since the lifestyle changes were minor—a 5 to 10 percent reduction in body weight and an exercise program of walking thirty minutes per day.

New studies are ongoing to see if the TZD class of oral agents (Avandia or Actos) will produce the same results, and if the drug metformin combined with lifestyle changes will produce even better results. Prevention is cheaper and certainly more healthy than treatment.

Update for Management of Type 1 and Type 2 Diabetes

The attitude toward the management of Type 1 diabetes, and to a lesser extent Type 2 diabetes, has been greatly changed by the Diabetes Control and Complications Trial (DCCT), which has shown conclusively that we need to obtain and maintain a high degree of control in order to prevent complications of diabetes. This has resulted in a great impetus to develop new methods of management. New dietary regimens or methodologies are being searched for and researched in order to improve control. These include carbohydrate counting and the point system. Carbohydrate counting is in fact a modification of the point system. But, to date, no scientific study has noted one approach to dietary therapy to be more beneficial than another.

However, techniques for really good control in keeping with the DCCT focus and principles have been developed. They are:

1. The care of the individual with diabetes by a specially trained team that is educated and experienced in the management of Type 1 diabetes,
2. The education of the patient in all aspects of diabetes, including principles of self-management, so that the patient can become empowered to take responsibility for his or her own care,
3. The use of a flexible dietary program that will match the insulin administration,
4. The use of a flexible multidose insulin regimen that can be modified to fit the various lifestyles of individuals with diabetes.

These are the principles that have guided the development of methodologies for managing Type 1 diabetes.

The DCCT study has proven beyond a doubt that blood sugar needs to be controlled in order to prevent the complications of the disease. But this study involved only people with Type 1 diabetes. What about Type 2 diabetes? Several studies have now been done to prove the same thing for Type 2 diabetes. The best of these studies is the United Kingdom Prospective Diabetes Study, or UKPDS. The study was discussed in an earlier chapter and will not be further discussed except to say again that the study is conclusive that control of blood sugar and blood pressure will prevent the complications of diabetes. This points up again the need for diabetes education, self-monitoring of blood sugar, and involvement of the diabetic in the day-to-day management of the disease, whether it is Type 1 or Type 2. This need for good control may lead to more persons going on insulin sooner than before, but this is a small price to pay for good health. New oral agents have been and are being developed to help keep people in good control without insulin, but what is most important is good control, not the tools we use to get the good control. Don't be afraid to use whatever tool or tools work for you and assist your doctor and educator in finding the proper tools by supplying the needed data (i.e., your daily blood sugars). Drugs can be combined in a variety of ways to effect good control. One, two, or even three drugs at a time can be used with or without a variety of insulin schedules to accomplish your goal: a long, healthy, productive life free of the complications of diabetes mellitus.

There are a number of drugs being developed to work in association with lowering your blood sugar to assist you in a better life. Some of these drugs are to regulate the emptying of the stomach, either to slow it down or to speed it up. There are also drugs being developed to slow, prevent, or reverse various complications. Unfortunately, many of the drugs tested so far are quite toxic, but the work goes on to develop better and less toxic drugs for these purposes. We hope that other technologies such as insulin that can be inhaled, taken orally, or absorbed through the skin; implantable sensors; bloodless meters; and others will soon be available. Until they are, it is very important that you use the tools available to maintain as good control as possible in order to prevent complications and to benefit from these new developments when they become available.

All this has led to the need for more blood-glucose self-monitoring in people with Type 2 diabetes so that these various medications can be individualized to meet the specific needs of these people as their needs change. Without blood-glucose self-monitoring and education, medication cannot be tailored to the needs of the individual, and the kind of control necessary to meet the standards of the DCCT and the UKPDS cannot be obtained. Therefore, it is our belief that all diabetic patients should be well educated and doing blood-glucose self-monitoring.

Funding for Research

Besides the National Institutes of Health, the major "funders" of diabetes research are the American Diabetes Association (ADA) and the Juvenile Diabetes Foundation. Still, the funds are not enough to support the many new ideas that are submitted for funding purposes. Funds are needed for salaries, equipment, supplies, and the paperwork involved in reporting and sharing information from investigator to investigator, and from the research centers to the public. Training funds are needed to develop the researchers of tomorrow. By the time a physician or other scientist completes the necessary research preparation, most of the funds have been used up.

For the physician, an offer of a medical practice often takes the place of research work so that he or she can have enough of an income to repay school debts and support a family.

Research training programs need supplies and equipment. Sometimes this equipment needs to be constructed to meet the researchers' guidelines (for example, in the case of the implantable artificial pancreas, no equipment was available to proceed with such an idea, so the machine had to be made from the ground up).

To aid research efforts, talk with your legislators and encourage an increase in funding for diabetes research. The ADA can supply you with statistics sheets of diabetes facts and comparisons of funding with other diseases that you can present to your congresspersons to help them understand the need for increased funding to eradicate this disease (for example, diabetes takes 15 percent of the national health dollar while AIDS takes only 3 percent, but AIDS gets 15 percent of the federal research dollars and diabetes gets only 1 percent). Support your diabetes association and their fund-raising efforts, and aid them in their efforts to alert the public to the dangers of diabetes and the need for research support.

The need for research into diabetes will be with us until the disease has finally been conquered. At present, education and knowledge are our best weapons. The more you, as an individual, keep yourself fit by following your program, the better able you will be to benefit from new research. And the more you share your ideas on the prevention, cure, or treatment of the disease with health professionals or diabetes associations, the more you will be helping to make diabetes mellitus a disease of the past.

Appendix A

Food Questionnaire

Phone: _____ Physician: _____

Name: _____ Date of birth: _____

Address: _____ Spouse: _____

How much milk do you drink per day? _____

Do you use butter? ☐ Margarine? ☐

If you use bread, what kind? White ☐ Whole grain ☐

If you use tortillas, what kind? Flour ☐ Corn ☐

If you use rice, what kind? White ☐ Brown ☐

Do you use kosher foods? Always ☐ Sometimes ☐ Never ☐

How many times per week do you eat the following foods?

Food	Never	Four or More	Daily	Serving Size
Hard cheese	_____	_____	_____	_____ Slices
Eggs	_____	_____	_____	_____ Whole
Steak, hamburger, pork chops, etc.	_____	_____	_____	_____ Ounces
Cold cuts, hot dogs, sausages, or luncheon meats	_____	_____	_____	_____ Pieces/ Ounces
Pizza	_____	_____	_____	_____ Pieces
Sweet rolls, doughnuts	_____	_____	_____	_____ Pieces
Deep-fat fried foods (French fries, etc.)	_____	_____	_____	_____ Pieces
Soda pop (diet or not)	_____	_____	_____	_____ Cups
Fruit drink (NOT fruit juice)	_____	_____	_____	_____ Cups
Alcoholic beverages, (beer, wine, whiskey, cocktails)	_____	_____	_____	_____ Cups Ounces
Milk shakes, ice cream, etc.	_____	_____	_____	_____ Cups
Candy	_____	_____	_____	_____ Pieces
Potato chips, other chips	_____	_____	_____	_____ Whole pieces
Crackers, pretzels	_____	_____	_____	_____ Whole pieces
Hot breads	_____	_____	_____	_____ Whole pieces

Food	Never	Four or More	Daily	Serving Size
Vegetables (dark green or deep yellow)	____	____	____	____ Cups
Citrus fruits (grapefruit, orange, tangerine, or tomato)	____	____	____	____ Cups
Potato	____	____	____	____ Whole
Sweet potato, yam	____	____	____	____ Whole
Corn, hominy	____	____	____	____ Cups
Other fruits and vegetables	____	____	____	____ Cups
Fish (including tuna)	____	____	____	____ Ounces
Chicken, turkey, other fowl	____	____	____	____ Ounces
Lean meat	____	____	____	____ Ounces
Cottage cheese or yogurt	____	____	____	____ Cups
Macaroni, noodles, spaghetti	____	____	____	____ Cups
Cereal, cooked	____	____	____	____ Cups
Cereal, dry	____	____	____	____ Cups
Corn bread, biscuits, bagels, muffins, waffles, pancakes	____	____	____	____ Whole pieces
Breads, buns, tortillas	____	____	____	____ Slices
Jelly, honey, jam, syrup, preserves	____	____	____	____ Tbsp
Tofu, nuts/seeds	____	____	____	____ Tbsp
Bacon, salt pork	____	____	____	____ Slices

Food	Never	Four or More	Daily	Serving Size
Peanut butter	_____	_____	_____	_____ Tbsp
Baked or cooked beans, (pinto, navy, butter, lima, lentil, split peas)	_____	_____	_____	_____ Cups
Soybeans	_____	_____	_____	_____ Cups
Salad dressing, mayonnaise	_____	_____	_____	_____ Tbsp
Rice, grits	_____	_____	_____	_____ Cups
Popcorn	_____	_____	_____	_____ Cups
Catsup	_____	_____	_____	_____ Tbsp
Molasses, sorghum	_____	_____	_____	_____ Tbsp
Chili	_____	_____	_____	_____ Cups
Sweetened gelatin or Popsicles	_____	_____	_____	_____ Cups/ Pieces
Pudding, custards, condensed milk	_____	_____	_____	_____ Cups
Cream	_____	_____	_____	_____ Tbsp
Gravy	_____	_____	_____	_____ Tbsp
Soup	_____	_____	_____	_____ Cups
Soup with milk	_____	_____	_____	_____ Cups
Olives, pickles	_____	_____	_____	_____ Pieces
Cocoa, chocolate	_____	_____	_____	_____ Cups/ Pieces
Chinese foods (chow mein, chop suey, etc.)	_____	_____	_____	_____ Cups
Italian foods (lasagna, spaghetti with meatballs, etc.)	_____	_____	_____	_____ Cups

Food	Never	Four or More	Daily	Serving Size
Tacos, tamales, enchiladas, etc.	_____	_____	_____	_____ Whole pieces
Macaroni and cheese	_____	_____	_____	_____ Cups

List other foods NOT listed above that you regularly eat:

_____

_____

_____

_____

_____

Circle what you use for seasoning foods:
salt in cooking, salt at table, monosodium glutamate, meat tenderizer, soy sauce, Tabasco, other:

_____

_____

_____

Circle the foods you like:
apricots, artichokes, avocados, bananas, bean sprouts, beets, bok choy, broccoli, brussels sprouts, cabbage, cantaloupe, carrots, green peppers, greens, mangoes, papayas, peas, radishes, raisins, sauerkraut, scallions, spinach, strawberries, swiss chard, turnips, watermelon, squash (kind) _____

Appendix B

Recommended Dietary Intakes

The development of Dietary Reference Intakes (DRIs; 2001) expands and replaces the series of Recommended Dietary Allowances (RDAs), which were published in 1941 by the Food and Nutrition Board of the National Academy of Sciences, and the Recommended Nutrient Intakes of Canada. Earlier reports (2, 3, and 4) in the series providing DRIs for some vitamins and other elements have been described previously, along with details on the framework and definitions of each category.

DRIs are reference values that are quantitative estimates of nutrient intakes to be used for planning and assessing diets for healthy people. They include RDIs as goals for intake by individuals but also present three new types of reference values (see Tables B.1 and B.2).

Definitions

Dietary Reference Intakes (DRIs): The average daily dietary intake level that is sufficient to meet the nutrient requirement of nearly all healthy individuals (97 to 98 percent) in a particular life stage and gender group.

Adequate Intake (AI): A recommended intake value based on observed or experimentally determined approximations or estimates of nutrient intake by a group (or groups) of healthy people that are assumed to be adequate; used when an RDI cannot be determined.

Tolerable Upper-Intake Level (UL): The highest level of daily nutrient intake that is likely to pose no risk of adverse health effects for almost all individuals in the general population. As intake increases above the UL, the potential risk of adverse effects increases.

Estimated Average Requirement (EAR): A daily nutrient intake value that is estimated to meet the requirement of half of the healthy individuals in a life stage and gender group.

Table B.1 Dietary Reference Intakes: Recommended Vitamin Intakes for Individuals
(Food and Nutrition Board, The Institute of Medicine National Academies)

Life Stage Group	Vitamin A (µg/d)[a]	Vitamin C (mg/d)	Vitamin D (µg/d)[b,c]	Vitamin E (mg/d)[d]	Vitamin K (µg/d)[a]	Thiamin (mg/d)	Riboflavin (mg/d)	Niacin (mg/d)[e]	Vitamin B6 (mg/d)	Folate (µg/d)[f]	Vitamin B12 (µg/d)[g]	Pantothenic Acid (mg/d)
Infants												
0–6 mo	400*	40.0*	5.0*	4.0*	2.0*	0.2*	0.3*	2.0*	0.1*	65*	0.4*	1.7*
7–12 mo	500*	50.0*	5.0*	5.0*	2.5*	0.3*	0.4*	4.0*	0.3*	80*	0.5*	1.8*
Children												
1–3y	300	15.0	5.0*	6.0	30.0*	0.5	0.5	6.0	0.5	150	0.9	2.0*
4–8y	400	25.0	5.0*	7.0	55.0*	0.6	0.6	8.0	0.6	200	1.2	3.0*
Males												
9–13y	600	45.0	5.0*	11.0	60.0*	0.9	0.9	12.0	1.0	300	1.8	4.0*
14–18y	900	75.0	5.0*	15.0	75.0*	1.2	1.3	16.0	1.3	400	2.4	5.0*
19–30y	900	90.0	5.0*	15.0	120.0*	1.2	1.3	16.0	1.3	400	2.4	5.0*
31–50y	900	90.0	5.0*	15.0	120.0*	1.2	1.3	16.0	1.3	400[h]	2.4	5.0*
51–70y	900	90.0	10.0*	15.0	120.0*	1.2	1.3	16.0	1.7	400	2.4[g]	5.0*
>70y	900	90.0	15.0*	15.0	120.0*	1.2	1.3	16.0	1.7	400	2.4[g]	5.0*
Females												
9–13y	600	45.0	5.0*	11.0	60.0*	0.9	0.9	12.0	1.0	300	1.8	4.0*
14–18y	700	65.0	5.0*	15.0	75.0*	1.0	1.0	14.0	1.2	400[h]	2.4	5.0*
19–30y	700	75.0	5.0*	15.0	90.0*	1.1	1.1	14.0	1.3	400	2.4	5.0*
31–50y	700	75.0	5.0*	15.0	90.0*	1.1	1.1	14.0	1.3	400	2.4	5.0*
51–70y	700	75.0	10.0*	15.0	90.0*	1.1	1.1	14.0	1.5	400	2.4[h]	5.0*
>70y	700	75.0	15.0*	15.0	90.0*	1.1	1.1	14.0	1.5	400	2.4[h]	5.0*
Pregnancy												
≤18y	750	80.0	5.0*	15.0	75.0*	1.4	1.4	18.0	1.9	600[i]	2.6	6.0*
19–30y	770	85.0	5.0*	15.0	90.0*	1.4	1.4	18.0	1.9	600[i]	2.6	6.0*
31–50y	770	85.0	5.0*	15.0	90.0*	1.4	1.4	18.0	1.9	600[i]	2.6	6.0*

Lactation

≤18y	1,200	115	5*	19	75*	1.4	1.6	17	2.0	500	2.8	7*
19–30y	1,300	120	5*	19	90*	1.4	1.6	17	2.0	500	2.8	7*
31–50y	1,300	120	5*	19	90*	1.4	1.6	17	2.0	500	2.8	7*

NOTE: This table (taken from the DRI reports; See www.nap.edu) presents Recommended Dietary Intakes (RDIs) and Adequate Intakes (AIs) followed by an asterisk (*). RDIs and AIs may both be used as goals for individual intake. RDIs are set to meet the needs of almost all (97 to 98 percent) individuals in a group. For healthy breastfed infants, the AI is the mean percentage of individuals covered by this intake.

[a]As retinal activity equivalents (RAEs). 1RAE = 1 µg retinol, 12 mg β-carotene, 24 α-carotene or 24 mg β-cryptoxanthin in foods. To calculate RAEs from REs of provitamin A carotenoids in foods, divide the REs by 2. For preformed vitamin A in foods or supplements and for provitamin A carotenoids in supplements, 1 RE = 1 RAE.

[b]Cholecalciferol. 1 mg cholecalciferol = 40 IU vitamin D.

[c]In the absence of adequate exposure to sunlight

[d]As a-tocopherol. A-tocopherol includes RRR-a-tocopherol, the only form of α-tocopherol that occurs naturally in foods, and the 2R-stereoisomeric forms of a-tocopherol (RRR-, RSR-, and RSS-a-tocopherol) that occur in fortified foods and supplements. It does not include the 2S-stereoisomeric forms of α-tocopherol (SRR-, SRS-, and SSS-α-tocopherol), also found in fortified foods and supplements.

[e]As niacin equivalents (NE). 1 mg of niacin = 60 mg of tryptopha; 0–6 months = preformed niacin (not NE).

[f]As dietary folate equivalents (DFE). 1 DFE = 1 mg food folate = 0.6 mg of folic acid from fortified food or as a supplement consumed with food = 0.5 mg of a supplement taken on an empty stomach.

[g]Because 10 to 30 percent of older people may malabsorb food-bound B₁₂, it is advisable for those older than 50 years to meet their RDI mainly by consuming food fortified with B₁₂ or a supplement containing B₁₂.

[h]In view of evidence linking folate intake with neural tube defects in the fetus, it is recommended that all women capable of becoming pregnant consume 400 mg from supplements or fortified foods in addition to intake of food folate from a varied diet.

[i]It is assumed that women will continue consuming 400 µg from supplements or fortified food until their pregnancy is confirmed and they enter prenatal care, which ordinarily occurs after the end of the periconceptional period—the critical time for formation of the neural tube.

Table B.2 Dietary Reference Intakes: Recommended Mineral Intakes for Individuals

(Food and Nutrition Board, The Institute of Medicine National Academies)

Life Stage Group	Calcium (mg/d)	Chromium (µg/d)	Copper (µg/d)	Fluoride (mg/d)	Iodine (µg/d)	Iron (mg/d)	Magnesium (mg/d)	Manganese (mg/d)	Molybdenum (µg/d)	Phosporous (mg/d)	Selenium (mg/d)	Zinc (mg/d)
Infants												
0–6 mo	210*	0.2*	200*	0.01*	110*	0.27	30*	0.003*	2*	100*	15*	2*
7–12 mo	270*	5.5*	220*	0.5*	130*	11	75*	0.6	3*	275*	20*	3*
Children												
1–3y	500*	11*	340	0.7*	90	7	80	1.2*	17	460	20	3
4–8y	800*	15*	440	1.0*	90	10	130	1.5*	22	500	30	5
Males												
9–13y	1,300*	25*	700	2.0*	120	8	240	1.9*	34	1,250	40	8
14–18y	1,300*	35*	890	3.0*	150	11	410	2.2*	43	1,250	55	11
19–30y	1,000*	35*	900	4.0*	150	8	400	2.3*	45	700	55	11
31–50y	1,000*	35*	900	4.0*	150	8	420	2.3*	45	700	55	11
51–70y	1,200*	30*	900	4.0*	150	8	420	2.3*	45	700	55	11
>70y	1,200*	30*	900	4.0*	150	8	420	2.3*	45	700	55	11
Females												
9–13y	1,300*	21*	700	2.0*	120	8	240	1.6*	34	1,250	40	8
14–18y	1,300*	24*	890	3.0*	150	15	360	1.6*	43	1,250	55	9
19–30y	1,000*	25*	900	3.0*	150	18	310	1.8*	45	700	55	8
31–50y	1,000*	25*	900	3.0*	150	18	320	1.8*	45	700	55	8
51–70y	1,200*	20*	900	3.0*	150	8	320	1.8*	45	700	55	8
>70y	1,200*	20*	900	3.0*	150	8	320	1.8*	45	700	55	8

Pregnancy											
≤18y	1,300*	29*	1,000	3*	220	27	400	2.0	50	1,250	60	13
19–30y	1,000*	30*	1,000	3*	220	27	350	2.0	50	700	60	11
31–50y	1,000*	30*	1,000	3*	220	27	360	2.0	50	700	60	11
Lactation											
≤18y	1,300*	44*	1,300	3*	290	10	360	2.6	50	1,250	70	14
19–30y	1,000*	45*	1,300	3*	290	9	310	2.6	50	700	70	14
31–50y	1,000*	45*	1,300	3*	290	9	320	2.6	50	700	70	12

NOTE: This table (taken from the DRI reports; See www.nap.edu) presents Recommended Dietary Intakes (RDIs) and Adequate Intakes (AIs) followed by an asterisk (*). RDIs and AIs may both be used as goals for individual intake. RDIs are set to meet the needs of almost all (97 to 98 percent) individuals in a group. For healthy breastfed infants, the AI is the mean percentage of individuals covered by this intake.

SOURCES: Dietary Reference Intakes for Calcium, Phosphorus, Magnesium, Vitamin D, and Fluoride (1997); Dietary Reference Intakes for Thiamin, Riboflavin, Niacin, Vitamin B₆, Folate, Vitamin B₁₂, Pantothenic Acid, Biotin, and Choline (1998); Dietary Reference Intakes for Vitamin C, Vitamin E, Selenium, and Carotenoids (2000) and Dietary Reference Intakes for Vitamin A, Vitamin K, Arsenic, Boron, Chromium, Copper, Iodine, Iron, Manganese, Molybdenum, Nickel, Silicon, Vanadium, and Zinc (2001). These reports may be accessed via www.nap.edu.

Appendix C

American Diabetes Association Exchange Lists*

The American Diabetes Association (ADA), in cooperation with the American Dietetic Association, promotes a program called *Carb Counting*. With this system, a point is given to ten to fifteen grams of carbohydrate and the person is educated as to how many points to have at meals and snack time. Although consideration is given to consuming nutritious protein and fats, the person's food intake is not limited except for carbohydrates consumed or if the person has a weight problem. The emphasis is on individual consultation with a registered dietitian.

The total amount of carbohydrate in the diet rather than the source seems to be the factor that influences after-meal blood-sugar levels. If table sugar (sucrose) is used as part of the meal plan, blood glucose is not necessarily affected. If used alone or added to the meal, it will account for elevated blood-sugar levels. This is not to say that one can freely use table sugar. Rather it means that sugar can be eaten in modest amounts as part of a balanced meal plan.

This approach to meal planning, the Carb Counting program, is quite useful. This is helpful for many people, but for growing children and others, recognition of total caloric intake and content in the basic meal plan is a must. Some people are still following the Exchange System, consuming food from specific groups for specific meals; others are

---

* Material on the following pages was adapted, with permission (1999), from the American Diabetes Association and the American Dietetic Association.

following the Point System (75 calories = 1 point), where food is distributed throughout the day to meet nutritional needs and the time action of medications. The Food Pyramid is also being used by itself or with the Point System. The Food Pyramid follows recommendations found in most meal plans: cereals, breads, rice, potatoes, and pasta form the base of the pyramid; the second level includes fruits and vegetables; the third includes dairy products, meat, fish, and eggs; and the top of the pyramid includes fats and sweets, with the admonition to use them sparingly (i.e., less than 30 percent of dietary calories should come from fat).

Weight loss is supported, but the focus on ideal body weight to height is not the goal as much as it was before. A mild to moderate weight loss of ten to twenty pounds has been shown to improve diabetes control. The goal is now focused on a healthy body weight and achieving desired blood-sugar and lipid (fat or cholesterol and triglyceride) levels. You may obtain a copy of the nutrition guidelines by contacting the Order Fulfillment Department at the American Diabetes Association's National Center at 1-800-232-3472.

When you eat, food is digested and much of it is changed into glucose, a sugar the body uses for fuel. The glucose is carried by the bloodstream to the individual cells of the body. The body produces a hormone called insulin that helps the glucose enter the cells. Normally, enough insulin is produced to allow the glucose in the blood to be absorbed by the cells, where it is used for energy. Insulin also helps the body to store extra glucose and fat for later use.

When you have diabetes, however, your body does not make enough, or any, insulin, or does not use it properly. Without insulin, your body cannot use the food you eat. The digested food, in the form of glucose, builds up in your blood. The cells can't get the energy they need because insulin isn't available to move the glucose into the cells. The symptoms of diabetes are caused by the high blood-glucose levels. People with diabetes may also have high blood-fat levels (cholesterol and triglycerides). Over time, higher-than-normal blood-glucose and blood-fat levels may cause serious long-term complications.

There are two major types of diabetes mellitus:

1. Type 1 diabetes (insulin-dependent [IDDM], juvenile onset)
2. Type 2 diabetes (non-insulin-dependent [NIDDM], adult onset)

People with Type 1 diabetes do not make insulin. When the body has no insulin and cannot use glucose for energy, it begins to burn fat. When fat is burned for energy, acid wastes called ketones are formed. The ketones build up in the blood and cause a serious condition called ketoacidosis. People with insulin-dependent diabetes must take insulin injections to avoid this life-threatening condition.

People with Type 2 diabetes make some or too much insulin, but either there is not enough or it does not work properly (insulin resistance). This type of diabetes can often be controlled through diet and exercise. Oral agents (diabetes pills) help some people to make more insulin, to use their own insulin better, or to block the uptake of carbohydrates from the intestine. Some people with Type 2 diabetes may need insulin injections to regulate their blood-glucose levels. Type 2 diabetes may also be found in children (more often in obese children).

Managing Diabetes with Food

The management of diabetes has three parts: food, activity, and medication (if needed). Food raises blood-glucose and blood-fat levels. Activity and medications (insulin or oral hypoglycemic agents) lower blood-glucose and blood-fat levels. A balance of these three parts leads to good management of diabetes. In this section, our focus will be on food.

The nutritional goals of diabetes management are appropriate blood-glucose and blood-fat levels. You will learn to balance the food you eat with your activity level and with the insulin in your body so that the levels of glucose and fats (cholesterol and triglycerides) in your blood stay as close to normal as possible. It is important to keep blood-glucose levels near normal to prevent problems that can result from too high a level (ketoacidosis or diabetic coma) or, if insulin is used, from too low a level (insulin reactions). It is important to match the amount of food you eat with the amount of insulin in your body, whether your body produces insulin (on its own or with the help of diabetes pills) or your insulin comes from injections. This will not only help you feel better (the symptoms of diabetes should disappear), but, more important, it may also help to reduce or prevent the complications of diabetes.

Blood-glucose monitoring can be useful in keeping track of your diabetes and can show the effects of certain foods or activities on your blood-glucose levels. You can measure your own blood glucose using a finger-stick device and test strip. Your monitoring record will help you match your meal plan to other aspects of your diabetes management.

It is also important to limit fat in your diet, because higher levels of blood fats are associated with heart disease. People with diabetes run a greater risk of developing heart disease than do other people.

Maintaining a Reasonable Weight

It is important to eat the right amount of calories to help you reach and stay at a reasonable body weight. The number of calories you need depends on your size, age, and activity level.

Eating too many calories causes weight gain, which will worsen diabetes and increase your risks for high blood pressure and heart disease. Your body makes and/or uses insulin best when you are at your desired weight.

Eating too few calories causes a different problem. Children and teens with diabetes must eat enough calories to grow properly. Pregnant and nursing women must eat enough calories to provide for proper development of their babies.

Exercise is very important, too. It is helpful in weight loss, and it is also good for your heart and blood vessels. You can increase your activity level by walking, biking, or just taking the stairs instead of an elevator. If you wish to begin an exercise training program, check with your health care team first.

Following Principles of Good Nutrition

It is important to eat a variety of foods each day. Your body works better if you eat a balanced diet that includes the right amounts of vitamins, minerals, carbohydrate, protein, and fat. Carbohydrate is the major source of energy. Protein builds muscle and tissue and provides some energy. Fat is the storage form of energy. Most foods contain a mixture of these. Carbohydrate, which has four calories per gram of weight, is found in starches, bread, fruit, vegetables, and milk. Protein also has four calories per gram of weight. Protein is found in meat and milk, and small amounts of it are found in starches, bread, and veg-etables. Fat is higher in calories, with nine calories per gram of weight. Fat is found in meat, dairy products, oils, and nuts. Insulin is needed to use carbohydrate, protein, and fat properly. Some principles of good nutrition follow:

Eat Less Fat. The average American adult eats too much fat. Too much fat may cause heart and blood vessel disease. Eat fish, poultry, and other lean meats. Watch your portion sizes with all meat—it's easy to eat too much. Eat fewer high-fat foods, such as cold cuts, bacon, nuts, gravy, salad dressing, margarine, and solid shortening. Drink skim or low-fat milk and eat less ice cream, butter, and cheese.

Eat More Carbohydrates (Starches and Breads), Especially Those High in Fiber. Carbohydrate foods are a good source of energy, vita-mins, and minerals. Fiber in foods may help to lower blood-glucose and blood-fat levels. All people should increase the amount of carbo-hydrate and fiber they eat. This can be done by eating more dried beans, peas, and lentils; more whole-grain breads, cereals, and crack-ers; and more fruits and vegetables. (Foods that are high in fiber will be noted later in this appendix with an asterisk [*].)

Eat Less Sugar. All people, not just those with diabetes, should eat less sugar. Sugar has lots of calories and no vitamins or minerals, and it causes cavities. Foods high in sugar include desserts (for example, frosted cake and pie), sugary breakfast foods, table sugar, honey, and syrup. One twelve-ounce can of a regular soft drink has nine teaspoons of sugar!

Use Less Salt. Most of us eat too much salt. The sodium in salt can cause the body to retain water, and in some people it may raise blood pressure. Try to use less salt in cooking and at the table. (Foods that are high in sodium, such as processed and convenience foods, will be noted later in this appendix with a pound sign [#].)

Use Alcohol in Moderation. It is best to avoid alcohol altogether, but if you like to have an alcoholic drink now and then, ask your die-titian how to work it into your meal plan. If you take insulin, it is important to eat food with your drink.

How Can I Accomplish These Goals?

Dietary counseling with a registered dietitian or a certified diabetes edu-cator knowledgeable in nutrition will help you to meet all these goals.

The first step is to talk to your dietitian, who will determine your present nutritional intake and then help you to work out your own nutritional plan. This plan will include the amount of carbohydrate you will choose to eat at specific times of the day, in relation to your nutritional needs of protein and fat, to round out your energy needs for your daily activity in line with the time action of your diabetes medication.

Are Meal Plans Different for Different Types of Diabetes?

Yes, they are. The goals of treatment are somewhat different for the two types of diabetes.

Type 1 Diabetes The most important nutrition principle for people with Type 1 diabetes is consistency. Meals should be eaten at about the same time each day. The amounts and types of food eaten at each meal should be about the same from day to day. This is important, because the food you eat is planned to balance your insulin injections and your activity. Your meal plan and the exchange lists can work together to regulate your blood-glucose levels. If your meal plan and your diabetes medication are out of balance, wide swings in blood-glucose levels can occur, and you may suffer from insulin reactions or from the symptoms of high blood-glucose levels.

Type 2 Diabetes Most people with Type 2 diabetes are overweight. Thus, the most important nutrition principle for people with this type of diabetes is weight control. You can lose weight by eating less food and increasing your exercise. It is still important to eat a balanced diet, even while losing weight. Your dietitian will help you to determine the number of calories you need and set weight goals, and will also give you tips to help you reach these goals.

Do I Have to Change the Way I Eat?

You may have to change the way you eat. Many people ask if they can eat the same foods as the rest of their family. The diabetes meal plan is not much different from the way everyone should eat. However, it is true that many people do not eat in such a healthful way. And it's very hard to change habits, especially about food. Just remember: Make changes gradually, set short-term goals, and reward yourself when you are successful.

To make your food intake work, you will need to consider how much you eat in relation to your activity, exercise, and diabetes medication. Serving sizes are very important to the success of your meal plan. If you eat too much food or too little food, your blood-glucose regulation and your weight will be affected. To help you estimate serving sizes accurately, you will need to measure or weigh your food for the first week or so, and again periodically as time goes on to see how you're doing. Suggestions for how to measure your serving sizes are included in the "Management Tips" section.

It is very important to see your dietitian regularly when you are first learning how to eat more nutritiously. Your food intake can be adjusted if it is not working for you. The only way to make it right is to see your dietitian and solve the problems.

Will This Meal Plan Always Be Right for Me?

What you eat and the way you plan to eat may need to be changed as time goes on. Changes in lifestyle (for example, those involving work, school, vacation, or travel) require adjustments in your meal plan. Your weight may change, your eating habits may change, or your activity may change—and any of these changes means you may need a new meal plan. As children grow they need more calories, and when they reach adulthood they need fewer. Check in with your dietitian regularly to review your meal plan, ask any questions you may have, and learn about new nutrition information. Regular nutrition counseling can help you make positive changes in your eating habits.

The Exchange Lists—Meal Planning

The reason for dividing food into six different groups is that foods vary in their carbohydrate, protein, fat, and calorie content. Each exchange list contains foods that are alike; each food choice on a list contains about the same amount of carbohydrate, protein, fat, and calories as the other choices on that list.

Table C.1 shows the amounts of nutrients in one serving from each exchange list. As you read the exchange lists, you will notice that one choice is often a larger amount of food than another choice from the same list. Because foods are so different, each food is measured or

Table C.1 Exchange List—Nutritional Amounts per Serving

	Carbohydrate (grams)	Protein (grams)	Fat (grams)	Calories	Calorie Points
I. Starch/Bread	15	3	trace	80	1
II. Meat					
Very Lean	–	7	0–1	35	½
Lean		7	3	55	¾
Medium-Fat	–	7	5	75	1
High-Fat	–	7	8	100	1½
III. Vegetable	5	2	–	25	½
IV. Fruit	15	–	–	60	1
V. Milk					
Skim	12	8	0–3	90	1
Low-Fat	12	8	5	120	1½
Whole	12	8	8	150	2
VI. Fat	–	–	5	45	½

weighed so that the amounts of carbohydrate, protein, fat, and calories are the same in each choice.

You will notice symbols beside some foods in the exchange groups. Foods that are high in fiber (3 grams or more per normal serving) are noted with an asterisk (*). High-fiber foods are good for you, and it is important to eat lots of these foods.

Foods that are high in sodium (400 milligrams or more of sodium per normal serving) are noted with a pound sign (#). As mentioned, it's a good idea to limit your intake of high-salt foods, especially if you have high blood pressure.

If you have a favorite food that is not included in any of these groups, ask your dietitian about it. That food can probably be worked into your meal plan, at least now and then.

I. Starch/Bread List (Equal to 1 Carb Point)

Each item in Table C.2 contains approximately 15 grams of carbohydrate, 3 grams of protein, a trace of fat, and 80 calories. Whole-grain products average about 2 grams of fiber per serving. Some foods are higher in fiber. Those foods that contain 3 or more grams of fiber per serving are identified with an asterisk (*).

Table C.2 Starch/Bread List

Cereals/Grains/Pasta

*Bran cereals, concentrated, such as Bran Buds, All Bran	⅓ cup
Bran cereals, flaked	½ cup
Bulgur (cooked)	½ cup
Cooked cereals	½ cup
Cornmeal (dry)	2½ tbsp
Grape Nuts	3 tbsp
Grits (cooked)	½ cup
Other ready-to-eat, unsweetened cereals	¾ cup
Pasta (cooked)	½ cup
Puffed cereal	1 cup
Rice, white or brown (cooked)	⅓ cup
Shredded wheat	½ cup
*Wheat germ	3 tbsp

Dried Beans/Peas/Lentils

*Beans and peas (cooked) such as kidney, white, split, black-eyed	⅓ cup
*Lentils (cooked)	⅓ cup
*Baked beans	¼ cup

Starchy Vegetables

*Corn	½ cup
*Corn on the cob, 1 ear	6" long
*Lima beans	½ cup
*Peas, green (canned or frozen)	½ cup
*Plantain	½ cup
Potato, baked 1 small	(3 oz)
Potato, mashed	½ cup
Squash, winter (acorn, butternut)	¾ cup
Yam, sweet potato (plain)	⅓ cup

*= 3 grams or more of fiber per serving

Bread

Bagel	½ (1 oz)
Bread sticks, crisp, 4" long	2 (⅔ oz)
Croutons, low fat	1 cup
English muffin	½
Frankfurter or hamburger bun	½ (1 oz)
Pita	4" across
Plain roll, small	1 (1 oz)
Raisin, unfrosted	1 slice
*Rye, pumpernickel,	1 slice (1 oz)
Tortilla, 6" across	1
White (including French, Italian)	1 slice (1 oz)
Whole wheat	1 slice

Crackers/Snacks

Animal crackers	8
Graham crackers, 2" square	3
Matzoh	¾ oz
Melba toast	5 slices
Oyster crackers	24
Popcorn, (popped, no fat added)	3 cups
Pretzels	¾ oz
Rye crisp, 2" × 3"	4
Saltine-type crackers	6
Whole wheat crackers, no fat added (crisp bread such as Finn, Kavli, Wasa)	2–4 (¾ oz)

Starchy Foods Prepared with Fat

(count as 1 starch/bread serving, plus fat serving)

Biscuit, 2" across	1
Chow mein noodles	½ cup
Corn bread, 2" cube	1 (2 oz)
Cracker, round butter type	6
French-fried potatoes (2–3" long)	1½ oz
Muffin, plain, small	1
Pancake, 4" across	2
Stuffing, bread (prepared)	¼ cup
Taco shell, 6" across	2
Waffle, 4" square	1
Whole-wheat crackers, fat added such as Triscuits)	4–6 (1 oz)

You can choose your starch exchanges from any of the items on this list. If you want to eat a starch food that is not on the list, the general rule is this:

½ cup of cereal, grain, or pasta = one serving
1 ounce of a bread product = one serving

Your dietitian can help you to be more exact.

II. Meat List (Equal to ±½ Carb Point)

Each serving of meat and substitutes on this list contains about seven grams of protein. The amount of fat and number of calories vary, depending on what kind of meat or substitute is chosen. The list is divided into four parts, based on the amount of fat and calories: very lean meat, lean meat, medium-fat meat, and high-fat meat. One ounce (one meat exchange) of each of these includes the nutrient amounts shown in Table C.3.

You are encouraged to include more lean and medium-fat meat, poultry, and fish in your meal plan (see Tables C.4 and C.5). This will help you to decrease your fat intake, which may help decrease your risk for heart disease. The items from the high-fat group are high in saturated fat, cholesterol, and calories (see Table C.6). You should limit your choices from the high-fat group to three times per week. Meat and substitutes do not contribute any fiber to your meal plan. Meats and meat substitutes that have 400 milligrams or more of sodium per exchange are indicated with the pound sign (#).

Table C.3 Meat List—Nutritional Amounts per Serving

	Carbohydrate (grams)	Protein (grams)	Fat (grams)	Calories	Calorie Points
Very lean	0	7	0–1	35	½
Lean	0	7	3	55	¾
Medium-Fat	0	7	5	75	1
High-Fat	0	7	8	100	1½

Tips

1. Bake, roast, broil, grill, or boil these foods rather than fry them with added fat.
2. Use a nonstick pan spray or a nonstick pan to brown or fry these foods.
3. Trim off visible fat before and after cooking.
4. Do not add flour, bread crumbs, coating mixes, or fat to these foods when preparing them.
5. Weigh meat after removing bones and fat and again after cooking. Three ounces of cooked meat are equal to about four ounces of raw meat. Some examples of meat portions are: 2 ounces meat (2 meat exchanges) = 1 small chicken leg or thigh, ½ cup cottage cheese or tuna; 3 ounces meat (3 meat exchanges) = 1 medium pork chop, 1 small hamburger, ½ of a whole chicken breast, 1 unbreaded fish fillet, or cooked meat, about the size of a deck of cards.
6. Restaurants usually serve prime cuts of meat, which are high in fat and calories.

Table C.4 Lean Meat and Substitutes

One exchange is equal to any one of the following items:

Beef	USDA Good or Choice grades of lean beef, such as round, sirloin, and flank steak; tenderloin; and chipped beef#	1 oz
Pork	Lean pork, such as fresh ham; canned, cured, or boiled ham#, Canadian bacon#, tenderloin	1 oz
Veal	All cuts are lean except for veal cutlets (ground or cubed)	1 oz
Poultry	Chicken, turkey, Cornish hen (without skin)	1 oz
Fish	All fresh and frozen fish	1 oz
	Crab, lobster, scallops, shrimp, clams (fresh 2 oz or canned in water#)	2 oz
	Oysters	6 med.
	Tuna# (canned in water)	¼ cup
	Herring (uncreamed or smoked)	1 oz
	Sardines (canned)	2 med.
Wild Game	Venison, rabbit, squirrel	1 oz
	Pheasant, duck, goose (without skin)	1 oz
Cheese	Any cottage cheese	¼ cup
	Grated parmesan	2 tbsp
	Diet cheese# (with fewer than 55 calories per ounce)	1 oz
Other	95% fat-free luncheon meat	1 oz
	Egg whites	3
	Egg substitutes (with fewer than 55 calories per ¼ cup)	¼ cup

= Foods high in sodium (400 mg or more sodium per serving)

Table C.5 Medium-Fat Meat and Substitutes

One exchange is equal to any one of the following items:

Beef	Most beef products fall into this category. Examples: all ground beef, roast (rib, chuck, rump), steak (cubed, Porterhouse, T-bone), and meat loaf.	1 oz
Pork	Most pork products fall into this category. Examples: chops, loin roast, Boston butt, cutlets.	1 oz
Lamb	Most lamb products fall into this category Examples: chops, leg, roast.	1 oz
Poultry	Chicken (with skin), domestic duck or goose (well drained of fat), ground turkey	1 oz
Fish	Tuna# (canned in oil and drained)	¼ cup
	Salmon# (canned)	¼ cup
Cheese	Skim or part-skim milk cheeses, such as:	
	Ricotta	¼ cup
	Mozzarella	1 oz
	Diet cheeses# (with 56–80 calories per ounce)	1 oz
Other	86% fat-free luncheon meat#	1 oz
	Egg (high in cholesterol, so limit to 3 per week)	1
	Egg substitutes (with 56–80 calories per ¼ cup)	¼ cup
	Tofu (2½" × 2¾" × 1")	4 oz
	Liver, heart, kidney, sweetbreads (high in cholesterol)	1 oz

= Foods high in sodium (400 mg or more sodium per serving)

Table C.6 High-Fat Meat and Substitutes

Remember, these items are high in saturated fat, cholesterol, and calories, and should be eaten only three times per week. One exchange is equal to any one of the following items:

Beef	Most USDA Prime cuts of beef, such as ribs, corned beef#	1 oz
Pork	Spareribs, ground pork, pork sausage# (patty or link)	1 oz
Lamb	Patties (ground lamb)	1 oz
Fish	Any fried fish product	1 oz
Cheese	All regular cheeses#, such as American, blue, Cheddar, Monterey, Swiss	1 oz
Other	Luncheon meat#, such as bologna, salami, pimiento loaf	1 oz
	Sausage#, such as Polish, Italian	1 oz
	Knockwurst, smoked	1 oz
	Bratwurst#	1 oz
	Frankfurter# (turkey or chicken)	1 frank
	Peanut butter (contains unsaturated fat)	1 tbsp

Count as one high-fat meat plus one fat exchange:

	Frankfurter# (beef, pork, or combination)	1 frank

= Foods high in sodium (400 mg or more sodium per serving)

III. Vegetable List (Equal to ½ Carb Point or Free)

Each vegetable serving in Table C.7 contains about 5 grams of carbohydrate, 2 grams of protein, and 25 calories. Vegetables contain 2 to 3 grams of dietary fiber. Vegetables that contain 400 mg of sodium per serving are identified with a pound sign (#).

Vegetables are a good source of vitamins and minerals. Fresh and frozen vegetables have more vitamins and less added salt. Rinsing canned vegetables will remove much of the salt.

Table C.7 Vegetable List

Unless otherwise noted, the serving size for vegetables (one vegetable exchange) is:

½ cup of cooked vegetables or vegetable juice
1 cup of raw vegetables

Artichoke (½ medium)
Asparagus
Beans (green, wax, Italian)
Bean sprouts
Beets
Broccoli
Brussels sprouts
Cabbage, cooked
Carrots
Cauliflower
Eggplant
Greens (collard, mustard, turnip)
Kohlrabi
Leeks

Mushrooms, cooked
Okra
Onions
Pea pods
Peppers (green)
Rutabaga
Sauerkraut#
Spinach, cooked
Summer squash (crookneck)
Tomato (one large)
Tomato/vegetable juice#
Turnips
Water chestnuts
Zucchini, cooked

Starchy vegetables such as corn, peas, and potatoes are found on the Starch/Bread List. For "free" vegetables (i.e., fewer than ten calories per serving), see the Free Foods List.

= Foods high in sodium (400 mg or more sodium per serving)

IV. Fruit List (Equal to 1 Carb Point)

Each item in Table C.8 contains about 15 grams of carbohydrate and 60 calories. Fresh, frozen, and dry fruits have about 2 grams of fiber per serving. Fruits that have 3 or more grams of fiber per serving have an asterisk (#). Fruit juices contain very little dietary fiber.

The carbohydrate and calorie contents for a fruit serving are based on the usual serving of the most commonly eaten fruits. Eat fresh fruits or frozen or canned fruits with no sugar added. Whole fruit is more filling than fruit juice and may be a better choice for those who are trying to lose weight.

Table C.8 Fruit List

Unless otherwise noted, the serving size for one fruit serving is:

½ cup of fresh fruit or fruit juice
¼ cup of dried fruit

Fresh, Frozen, and Unsweetened Canned Fruit

Apples (raw, 2" across)	1
Applesauce, (unsweetened)	½ cup
Apricots (canned, 4 halves)	½ cup
Banana (9" long)	½
Blackberries (raw)	¾ cup
Blueberries (raw)	¾ cup
Cantaloupe (5" across)	⅓
(cubes)	1 cup
Cherries	
(large, raw)	12 whole
(canned)	½ cup
Figs (raw, 2" across)	2
Fruit cocktail (canned)	½ cup
Grapefruit (medium)	½
(segments)	¾ cup
Grapes (small)	15
Honeydew melon (medium)	⅛
(cubes)	1 cup
Kiwi (large)	1
Mandarin oranges	¾ cup
Mango (small)	½
Nectarines (2½" across)	1
Orange (2½" across)	1
Papaya	1 cup
Peach (2¾" across)	¾ cup
Peaches (canned, 2 halves)	1 cup
Pear (½ large)	1 small

Pear (canned, 2 halves)	½ cup
Persimmon (medium, native)	2
Pineapple (raw)	¾ cup
Pineapple (canned)	⅓ cup
Plum (raw, 2" across)	2
*Pomegranate	½
*Raspberries (raw)	1 cup
*Strawberries (raw, whole)	1¼ cups
Tangerine (2½" across)	2
Watermelon (cubes)	1¼ cups

*Dried Fruit

*Apples	4 rings
*Apricots	7 halves
Dates (medium)	2½
*Figs	1½
*Prunes (medium)	3
Raisins	2 tbsp

Fruit Juice

Apple juice/cider	½ cup
Cranberry juice cocktail	⅓ cup
Grapefruit juice	½ cup
Grape juice	⅓ cup
Orange juice	½ cup
Pineapple juice	½ cup
Prune juice	⅓ cup

*= 3 grams or more of fiber per serving

Table C.9 Milk List—Nutritional Amounts per Serving

	Carbohydrate (grams)	Protein (grams)	Fat (grams)	Calories
Skim	12	8	trace	90
Low-Fat	12	8	5	120
Whole	12	8	8	150

V. Milk List (Equal to 1 Carb Point)

Each serving of milk or milk products in Table C.9 contains about 12 grams of carbohydrate and 8 grams of protein. The amount of fat in milk is measured in percent of butterfat. The calories vary depending on the kind of milk chosen. The list is divided into three parts, based on the amount of fat and calories: skim/very low-fat milk, low-fat milk, and whole milk. One serving (one milk exchange) of each of these is shown. See Table C.10 for specific serving sizes.

Milk is the body's main source of calcium, the mineral needed for growth and repair of bones. Yogurt is also a good source of calcium. Yogurt and many dry or powdered milk products have different amounts of fat. If you have questions about a particular item, read the label to find out the fat and calorie content.

Milk can be drunk or added to cereal or other foods. Many tasty dishes, such as sugar-free pudding, are made with milk (see the Combination Foods list). Add life to plain yogurt by adding one of your fruit servings to it.

Table C.10 Milk List

Skim and Very Low Fat Milk

Skim milk	1 cup
½% milk	1 cup
1% milk	1 cup
Low-Fat buttermilk	1 cup
Evaporated skim milk	½ cup
Dry nonfat milk	⅓ cup
Plain nonfat yogurt	8 oz

Low-Fat Milk

2% milk	1 cup
Plain low-fat yogurt (with added nonfat milk solids)	8 oz

Whole Milk

The whole-milk group has much more fat per serving than the skim and low-fat groups. Whole milk has more than 3¼% butterfat. Try to limit your choices from the whole-milk group as much as possible.

Whole milk	1 cup
Evaporated whole milk	½ cup
Whole milk plain yogurt	8 oz

VI. Fat List

Each serving in Table C.11 contains about 5 grams of fat and 45 calories.

The foods on the fat list contain mostly fat, although some items may also contain a small amount of protein. All fats are high in calories and should be carefully measured. Everyone should modify fat intake by eating unsaturated fats instead of saturated fats. The sodium content of these foods varies widely. Check the label for sodium information.

Table C.11 Fat List

Unsaturated Fats

Avocado, medium	⅛
Margarine	1 tsp
# Margarine, diet	1 tbsp
Mayonnaise	1 tsp
# Mayonnaise (reduced-calorie)	1 tbsp
Nuts and Seeds:	
Almonds, dry roasted	6
Cashews, dry roasted	1 tbsp
Pecans	2
Peanuts (small)	20
(large)	10
Walnuts	2 whole
Other nuts	1 tbsp
Seeds (except pumpkin, pine nuts, sunflower (shelled)	1 tbsp
Pumpkin seeds	2 tbsp
Oil (corn, cottonseed, safflower, soybean, sunflower, olive, peanut)	1 tbsp
# Olives (small)	10
large)	5
Salad dressing, all varieties, regular	1 tbsp
Salad dressing, mayonnaise-type reduced-calorie	1 tbsp
Salad dressing, mayonnaise-type regular	2 tbsp
Salad dressing, reduced-calorie (2 tbsp of low-calorie dressing is a free food)	2 tbsp

Saturated Fats

Butter	1 tsp
# Bacon	1 slice
Chitterlings	½ oz
Coconut, shredded	2 tbsp
Coffee whitener, liquid	2 tbsp
Coffee whitener, powder	4 tsp
Cream (light, coffee, table)	2 tbsp
Cream, sour	2 tbsp
Cream (heavy, whipping)	1 tbsp
Cream cheese	1 tbsp
# Salt pork	¼ oz

= 400 mg or more of sodium if more than one or two servings are eaten

Free Foods

A free food (see Table C.12) is any food or drink that contains fewer than 20 calories per serving. You can eat as much as you want of items that have no serving size specified. You may eat two or three servings per day of those items that have a specific serving size. Be sure to spread them out through the day.

Table C.12 Free Foods

Drinks		Salad Greens	
#Bouillon or broth without fat		Endive	
Bouillon, low-sodium		Escarole	
Carbonated drinks, sugar-free		Lettuce	
Carbonated water		Romaine	
Club soda		Spinach	
Cocoa powder, unsweetened	1 tbsp		
Coffee/tea		**Sweets**	
Drink mixes, sugar-free		Candy, hard, sugar-free	
Tonic water, sugar-free		Gelatin, sugar-free	
		Gum, sugar-free	
Fruits and Vegetables		Jam/jelly, sugar-free	2 tsp
Cranberries, unsweetened	½ cup	Pancake syrup, sugar-free	1–2 tbsp
Rhubarb, unsweetened	½ cup	Sugar substitutes	
Vegetables, raw	1 cup	(saccharin, aspartame)	
Cabbage		Whipped topping	2 tbsp
Celery			
*Chinese cabbage		**Condiments**	
Cucumber		Catsup	1 tbsp
Green onion		Horseradish	
Hot peppers		Mustard	
Mushrooms		#Pickles, dill, unsweetened	
Radishes		Salad dressing, low-calorie	2 tbsp
*Zucchini		Taco sauce	1 tbsp
		Vinegar	
*= 3 grams or more per serving			
# = 400 mg or more of sodium per serving		**Nonstick pan spray**	

Seasonings

Seasonings can be very helpful in making foods taste better (see Table C.13). But be careful how much sodium you use. Read labels to help you choose seasonings that do not contain sodium or salt.

Table C.13 Seasonings

Basil (fresh)	Lemon pepper
Celery seeds	Lime
Chili powder	Lime juice
Chives	Mint
Cinnamon	Onion powder
Curry	Oregano
Dill	Paprika
Flavoring extracts (vanilla, almond,	Pepper
walnut, butter, peppermint, lemon, etc.)	Pimento
Garlic	#Soy sauce
Garlic powder	Soy sauce, low sodium ("lite")
Herbs	Spices
Hot pepper sauce	Wine, used in cooking (¼ cup)
Lemon	Worcestershire sauce
Lemon juice	

= 400 mg or more of sodium per serving

Combination Foods

Much of the food we eat is mixed together in various combinations. These combination foods do not fit into only one exchange list. It can be quite hard to tell what is in a certain casserole dish or baked food item. Table C.14 includes average values for some typical combination foods to help you fit these foods into your meal plan. Ask your dietitian for information about any other foods you'd like to eat. The American Diabetes Association/American Dietetic Association Family Cookbooks and the *American Diabetes Association Holiday Cookbook* have many recipes and further information about many foods, including combination foods. Check your library or local bookstore.

Table C.14 Combination Foods

(15 grams = 1 Carb Point)
(75 calories = 1 Calorie Point

Food	Amount	Exchanges	Carb Points	Calorie Points
Casserole, homemade	1 cup (8 oz)	2 medium-fat meats 2 starches, 1 fat	2	4½
#Cheese pizza, thin crust	¼ of a 15-oz pizza or a 10' pizza	1 medium-fat meat, 2 starches, 1 fat	2	3½
*#Chili with beans, commercial	1 cup (8 oz)	1 medium-fat meat, 2 starches, 2 fats	2	4
*#Chow mein (without noodles or rice)	2 cups (16 oz)	2 lean meats, 1 starch, 2 vegetables	2	3½
#Macaroni and cheese	1 cup (8 oz)	1 medium-fat meat, 2 starches, 2 fats	2	4
Soups				
*#Bean	1 cup (8 oz)	1 lean meat, 1 starch, 1 vegetable	1½	2¼
#Chunky, all varieties	10¾-oz can	1 medium-fat meat, 1 starch, 1 vegetable	1½	2½
#Cream (made with water)	1 cup (8 oz)	1 starch, 1 fat	1	1½
#Vegetable or broth	1 cup (8 oz)	1 starch	1	1
Other				
*#Spaghetti and meatballs (canned)	1 cup (8 oz)	1 medium-fat meat, 1 fat, 2 starches	2	3½
Sugar-free pudding (made with skim milk)	½ cup	1 starch	1	1
If beans are used as a meat substitute:				
*Dried beans, peas, lentils	1 cup (cooked)	1 lean meat, 2 starches	2	2¾

= 400 mg or more of sodium if more than one serving is consumed

* = 3 grams or more per serving

Table C.15 Occasional Foods

(15 grams = 1 Carb Point
(75 calories = 1 Calorie Point

Food	Amount	Exchanges	Carb Points	Calorie Points
Angel-food cake	¹⁄₁₂ cake	2 starches	2	2
Cake, no icing (3" square)	¹⁄₁₂ cake	2 starches, 2 fats	2	3
Cookies (1¾" across)	2 small	2 starches, 2 fats	2	3
Frozen fruit yogurt	⅓ cup	1 starch	1	1
Gingersnaps	3	1 starch	1	1
Granola	¼ cup	1 starch, 1 fat	1	1½
Granola bars	1 small	1 starch, 1 fat	1	1½
Ice cream, any flavor	½ cup	1 starch, 2 fats	1	2
Ice milk, any flavor	½ cup	1 starch, 1 fat	1	1½
Sherbet, any flavor	¼ cup	1 starch	1	1
#Snack chips, all varieties	1 oz	1 starch, 2 fats	1	2
Vanilla wafers	6 small	1 starch, 1 fat	1	1½

= 400 mg or more of sodium per serving if more than one serving is consumed

Occasional Foods

Moderate amounts of some foods can be used in your meal plan, in spite of their sugar or fat content, as long as you can maintain blood-glucose control. Table C.15 lists average values for some of these foods. Because they are concentrated sources of carbohydrate, you will notice that the portion sizes are very small. Check with your dietitian for advice on how often and when you can eat them.

Management Tips

Here are some tips that can help you to change the way you eat.

Make changes gradually
Don't try to do everything all at once. It may take longer to accomplish your goals, but the changes you make will be permanent.

Set Short-Term, Realistic Goals
If weight loss is your goal, try to lose two pounds in two weeks, not twenty pounds in one week. Walk two blocks at first, not two miles. Success will come more easily, and you'll feel good about yourself.

Reward Yourself
When you achieve your short-term goal, do something special for yourself—go to a movie, buy a new shirt, read a book, visit a friend.

Measure Foods
It is important to estimate the serving sizes of food. You can train your eye better by measuring all the food you are served. You can do this by measuring all the food you eat for a week or so. Measure liquids with a measuring cup. Some solid foods (such as tuna, cottage cheese, and canned fruits) can also be measured with a measuring cup. Measuring spoons are used for measuring smaller amounts of other foods (such as oil, salad dressing, and peanut butter). A scale can be very useful for measuring almost anything, especially meat, poultry, and fish. All food should be measured or weighed after cooking.

Some food you buy uncooked will weigh less after you cook it. This is true of most meats. Starches often swell in cooking, so a small amount of uncooked starch will become a much larger amount of cooked food. Table C.16 shows some of the changes.

Read Food Labels
Remember, dietetic does not mean diabetic! When you see the word *dietetic* on a food label, it means that something has been changed or replaced. It may have less salt, less fat, or less sugar. It does not mean that the food is sugar-free or calorie-free. Some dietetic foods may be useful. Those that contain 20 calories or less per serving may be eaten up to three times a day as free foods.

Table C.16 Uncooked to Cooked, Starch Changes

Starch Group	Uncooked	Cooked
Oatmeal	3 level tbsp	½ cup
Cream of wheat	2 level tbsp	½ cup
Grits	3 level tbsp	½ cup
Rice	2 level tbsp	⅓ cup
Spaghetti	¼ cup	½ cup
Noodles	⅓ cup	½ cup
Macaroni	¼ cup	½ cup
Dried beans	3 tbsp	⅓ cup
Dried peas	3 tbsp	⅓ cup
Lentils	2 tbsp	⅓ cup
Meat Group		
Hamburger	4 oz	3 oz
Chicken	1 small drumstick	1 oz
	½ of whole breast	3 oz

Using Carb Counting

There is simple counting and then, with consideration of protein in the diet, there is more complex carb counting. The American Diabetes Association has booklets that can graduate you from the simpler to the more complex program. Recognize that you can control neither blood glucose levels nor weight if only carbohydrate intake is controlled and you eat all the protein and fat you wish.

All the answers on the "right" approach to meal planning are not in. During the National American Diabetes Association meeting and at the national meeting of the American Association of Diabetes Educators, a panel of nutrition specialists came to this same conclusion. Various programs have merits, but the meal plan to end all meal planning is yet to come.

Know Your Sweeteners

Two types of sweeteners are on the market: those with calories and those without calories. Sweeteners with calories (such as fructose, sorbitol, and mannitol) may cause cramping and diarrhea when used in large amounts. Remember, these sweeteners do have calories, which can add up. Sweeteners without calories include saccharin and aspartame (Equal, Nutrasweet) and may be used in moderation.

If You Have Type 1 Diabetes

Plan for Sick Days

Before you become ill with the flu or a cold, ask your doctor, dietitian, or nurse for a special sick-day plan. When you are ill, it is important to do the following:

- Take your usual insulin dose.
- Test your blood glucose regularly, and check your urine for ketones.
- If you can't keep regular food down, try drinking small sips of regular soft drinks, sweetened tea, sweetened gelatin, Popsicles, fruit juice, or sherbet. (Call your doctor immediately if you can't keep any food down.)
- Drink lots of liquids.

Prepare for Insulin Reactions

If you have symptoms of low blood glucose, test your blood to find out your blood-glucose level. Be sure to carry something with you at all times to treat low blood glucose (for example, glucose tablets or hard candy).

Plan for Exercise

You may need to make some changes in your meal plan or insulin dose when you begin an exercise program. Check with your dietitian or doctor about this. Be sure to carry some form of carbohydrate with you to treat low blood glucose (for example, dried fruit or glucose tablets). Additional information on these topics is available from your dietitian or other health professional.

Glossary of Nutrition–Related Terms

Alcohol—An ingredient in a variety of beverages, including beer, wine, liqueurs, cordials, and mixed or straight drinks. Pure alcohol itself yields about 7 calories per gram, of which more than 75 percent is available to the body.

Calorie—A unit used to express the energy value of food. Calories come from carbohydrates, proteins, fats, and alcohol. (75 calories = 1 point)

Carbohydrate—One of the three major energy sources in foods. The most common carbohydrates are sugar and starches. Carbohydrates yield about 4 calories per gram. Carbohydrates are found in foods from the milk, vegetable, fruit, and starch/bread exchange lists. Fifteen grams of carbohydrate equals one carb point and one calorie point.

Cholesterol—A fatlike substance normally found in blood. A high level of cholesterol in the blood has been shown to be a major risk factor for developing heart disease. Dietary cholesterol is found in all animal products, but it is especially high in egg yolks and organ meats. Eating foods high in dietary cholesterol and saturated fat tends to raise the level of blood cholesterol. Foods of plant origin, such as fruits, vegetables, grains, and legumes, contain no cholesterol. Cholesterol is found in milk, meat, and fat-containing foods.

Dietitian—A registered dietitian (R.D.) is recognized by the medical profession as the primary provider of nutritional care, education, and counseling. The initials "R.D." after a dietitian's name ensure that he or she has met the standards of the American Dietetic Association. Look for this credential when you seek advice on nutrition.

Exchange—Foods grouped together on a list according to similarities in food values. Measured amounts of foods within the group may be used as trade-offs in planning meals. All of the exchanges in a group contain approximately equal amounts of carbohydrate, protein, fat, and calories. (½ calorie point.

Fat—One of the three energy sources in food. A concentrated source of calories, with about 9 calories per gram. Fat is found in foods such as meat, nonskim milk based products, butter, margarine, and salad dressings. One gram of fat equals ½ calorie point.

Fat, saturated—This fat tends to raise blood-cholesterol levels. It comes primarily from animals and is often hard at room temperature. Examples of saturated fats are butter, lard, meat fat, solid shortening, palm oil, and coconut oil.

Fat, unsaturated—This type of fat—monounsaturated in particular—tends to lower blood-cholesterol levels. Polyunsaturated fat neither raises nor lowers them. Unsaturated fat comes from plants and is usually liquid at room temperature. Examples of monounsaturated fats are olive, canola, and avocado oils, while examples of polyunsaturated fats are corn, cottonseed, sunflower, safflower, and soybean oils.

Fiber—An indigestible part of certain foods. Fiber is important in the diet as roughage, or bulk. Fiber is found in foods from the starch/bread, vegetable, and fruit exchange lists.

Fiber, insoluble—Found in foods such as wheat bran and other whole grains; has poor water-holding capability. It appears to speed the passage of foods through the stomach and intestines, and it increases fecal bulk. This type of fiber probably does not affect glycemic response or arteriosclerosis.

Fiber, soluble—Has high water-holding capability and turns to gel during digestion, which slows digestion and the rate of nutrition absorption from the stomach and intestine. This type of fiber is found in oat bran, pectins (in fruits and vegetables), and various "gums" that are found in nuts, seeds, and legumes such as beans, lentils, and peas. This type of fiber may play a role in smoothing out the glycemic response of foods and in reducing the likelihood of arteriosclerosis.

Glycosylated hemoglobin—A test that gives information about blood-glucose levels during the preceding one to two months. When blood glucose is above normal, the glucose attaches to the protein (or hemoglobin) in red blood cells. These cells last for about 120 days and can be measured.

Gram—A unit of mass and weight in the metric system. One ounce is equal to about 30 grams.

Insulin—A hormone made by the body that helps the body use food. Also, a commercially prepared injectable substance used by people who do not make enough of their own insulin.

Ketoacidosis—An increase in ketones in the blood, causing the body's acid balance to tip. An emergency situation that may result in coma and death if untreated.

Ketone—An acid that forms in the body when fats are burned for energy.

Meal plan—A guide showing the types of foods to use in each meal and snack to control the distribution of carbohydrates, proteins, fats, and calories throughout the day.

Mineral—Substance essential in small amounts to build and repair body tissue and/or control functions of the body. Examples include calcium, iron, magnesium, phosphorus, potassium, sodium, and zinc.

Nutrient—Substance in food necessary for life. Carbohydrates, protein, fats, minerals, vitamins, and water are nutrients.

Nutrition—Combination of processes by which the body receives and uses the materials necessary for maintenance of functions, for energy, and for growth and renewal of its parts.

Protein—One of the three major nutrients in food. Protein provides about 4 calories per gram. Protein is found in milk and meats. Smaller amounts of protein may be found in vegetables and starches. (½ carb point; ¾, 1, 1½ calorie point)

Sodium—A mineral needed by the body to maintain life, found mainly as a component of salt. Many individuals need to cut down the amount of sodium (and salt) they eat to help control high blood pressure.

Starch—One of the two major types of carbohydrates. Foods consisting mainly of starch come from the starch/bread exchange list.

Sugar—One of the two major types of carbohydrates. Foods consisting mainly of simple sugars are those from the milk, vegetable, and fruit exchange lists. Other simple sugars include common table sugar and the sugar alcohols (sorbitol, mannitol, and others).

Triglycerides—A fat that the body makes from food and that is normally present in the blood. Excess weight or consumption of too much fat, alcohol, and sugar may increase the blood triglycerides to an unacceptably high level.

Type 1 diabetes—Insulin-dependent diabetes mellitus. Individuals with Type 1 diabetes are ketosis-prone and will develop ketoacidosis if they do not take insulin regularly.

Type 2 diabetes—Non-insulin-dependent diabetes mellitus. Individuals with Type 2 diabetes may or may not need to take insulin for better control of their blood-glucose levels; however, they are not ketosis-prone.

Vitamins—Substances found in food and needed in small amounts to assist in bodily processes and functions. These include vitamins A, D, E, B-complex, C, and K.

Appendix D

Meal Planning—
Points in Nutrition

Nutritionists are still looking for the right approach to entice people to eat nutritiously. In the summer of 2001, the American Diabetes Association and the American Association of Diabetes Educators both had a panel of experts discuss the pros and cons of each of the programs, based on the latest scientific information. Their conclusions were that the best program is still to be found and that the individualization needed may lead a person to choose one approach over another just because that approach seems to be better for him or her.

Dr. A. T. Woodyatt, the physician who developed the Total Available Glucose (TAG) system, was working with a Midwest, predominantly Polish-speaking population in the 1930s. He developed the Point System in order to teach "normal" nutrition. Points and symbols were given for calories, carbohydrate, protein, and fat-containing foods, along with some of the most commonly found vitamins and minerals (A, three different B vitamins, C, iron, and calcium). Virginia Stuckey, R.D., who worked for Dr. Woodyatt in the fifties, switched from teaching the Exchange System to teaching about the Point System. All of this was based on the responses of her clients and the professionals with whom she had contact.

Virginia Stuckey educated us about the Point System and we found, after trials using just carbohydrate or protein or fat points, that calorie points along with intensive nutrition education appeared to be the most flexible program we had encountered and still met the needs

215

of aiding in the process of controlling the blood-glucose levels of most of our population. Now we use calorie points corresponding with the Food Pyramid model for balanced nutrition. Using the common serving sizes, a bread, cereal, or other grain serving is one point. One ounce of meat is one point, unless it is fatty meat (1½ points) or, at the other extreme, very lean (¾ point). A fruit serving is one point, a vegetable serving of compact carbohydrate (such as potato or rice) is one point, and a less compact carbohydrate (such as green beans or squash) is ½ point. Skim milk and related products are one point per eight-ounce glass, while 2% milk is 1½ points and a glass of whole milk is 2 points. Anything in the fat group (such as a teaspoon of butter or margarine or a tablespoon of salad dressing) is equal to ½ point. Sweets can also be given a point value, but you are encouraged to eat such items infrequently and with or at the end of a meal or snack.

The preceding food choices list (see Table D.1) includes examples of food serving sizes and their point values. A key to abbreviations used is on the following page.

Free Foods
Lettuce, greens, small amounts of raw vegetables, beverages with 0 calories.

Decaffeinated beverages are preferred. Fruits are unsweetened. Vegetables have no added fat. Meats are baked or broiled.

c = cup	diam = diameter
oz = ounce	sq = square
tbsp = tablespoon	" = inch
tsp = teaspoon	

For more information, consult:

"Points in Your Favor"
Diabetes Education Center
Via Christi—St. Joseph Campus
3600 East Harry
Wichita, KS 67218
316-689-6080

Table D.1 Food Choices (Not a complete list)

Menu Items	Calorie Points*	Menu Items	Calorie Points*
Apple, 1–3" diam	1	Fish, 2 oz	1
Applesauce, ½ c	1	Grapes, 1 c	1
Apricots, 3 halves	½	Grapefruit	
Asparagus, ½ c	½	fresh, ½	½
Avocado, ½–3" diam	2	juice, 1 c	1
Bacon, 1 slice	½	Grape juice, 1 c	2
Bagel, 1–3" diam	2	Lamb, lean, 2 oz	1½
Banana, 1–9"	1½	Macaroni, 1 c	2
Beans		Mayonnaise, 1 tbsp	1½
baked, ½ c	2	Milk	
navy, ½ c	1½	2%, 1 c	1½
green, ½ c	0	skim, 1 c	1
Beef, lean, 1 oz	1	whole, 1 c	2
Beef stew, 1 c	3	Muffin, 3" diam	1½
Beer		Noodles, 1 c	3
lite, 12 oz	1½	Nuts	
regular, 12 oz	2	cashews, 6–8	1
Biscuit, 2" diam	1½	mixed, 8–12	1
Bran, 100%, ½ c	1½	walnuts, 8–10	1
Bran flakes, ½ c	1	Oatmeal, 1 c	2
Bread, 1 slice	1	Oils, 1 tbsp	1½
Broccoli, ⅔ c	½	Olives, 6	½
Brussels sprouts, 7–8	½	Onion, ½ c	½
Buns		Orange, 3" diam	1
hamburger or hot dog	1½	Orange juice, 1 c	1½
Butter, 1 pat	½	Pancake, 6" diam	2
Cabbage, ½ c	0	Peach, 3" diam	½
Cantaloupe, 1 c	1	Peanuts, 1 oz	2
Carrot, ½	0	Peanut butter, 2 tsp	1
Casserole, 1 c	5	Pear, 3" × 4"	1½
Cauliflower, ½ c	0	Peas, green, ½ c	1
Cheese, hard yellow, 1 oz	1½	Pepper, green, 1 large	½
Chicken, 1 oz	1	Pineapple (unsweetened)	
Cold cuts, 1 slice	1	canned, 1 c	2
Corn, ½ c	1	juice, 1 c	2
Corn bread, 2" sq	2½	Pita bread, 6" diam	2
Corn flakes, 1 c	1½	Plums, 1 medium	½
Cottage cheese, 4% fat, ½ c	1½	Popcorn, plain, 3 c	1
Cracker, 3 sq	½	Pork, lean, 1 oz	1
(standard-size saltine crackers)		Potatoes	
Cream		baked, 1 medium	2
half and half, 2 tbsp	½	chips, 2 oz	4
sour cream, 2 tbsp	½	French-fried, 4" strips	2
Croissant, 1	3	mashed, ½ c	1½
Egg, 1	1	Pretzels, 6 sticks	1
Fat (margarine, oil), 1 tsp	½	Prunes	
		canned, 5	1
		juice, 1 c	2½

* 75 calories = 1 point

Menu Items	Calorie Points*	Menu Items	Calorie Points*
Raisins, 2 tbsp	½	Sweet potato, 2" × 4"	3
Rice, 1 c	3	Tomato	
Roll, 2" diam	1	raw, 1 medium	½
Salad dressing,1 tbsp	1	juice, 1 c	½
Sauerkraut, ½ c	½	**Catsup, 2 tbsp	½
Spaghetti, 1 c	2	Veal, 2 oz	2
Spinach, 1 c	½	Waffle, 7" diam	3½
Squash, winter, ½ c	½	Watermelon, 1 c	½
Strawberries, 1 c	½	Yogurt, plain, 1 c	2

* 75 calories = 1 point

** Contains too much sugar

Appendix E

Restaurant Guide Food Choices

Menu Items	Calorie Points*	Menu Items	Calorie Points*
ARBY'S		*Breakfast*	
Arby's Sauce, 1 oz	½	**Croissant	
Arby's Sub (no dressing)	6½	Arby's Butter	3
Bac 'n' Cheddar Deluxe	7½	Bacon & Egg	5½
Beef 'n' Cheddar	6½	Ham & Swiss	4½
Chicken Breast Sandwich	8	Mushroom & Swiss	4½
Chicken Club Sandwich	8½	Sausage & Egg	7
Chicken Salad Croissant	6	**ASIAN FOOD ESTIMATES**	
French Dip	5	Almond Chicken	7
French Fries (2½ oz)	4	Broccoli Beef, 1½ c	6
Ham 'n' Cheese	6½	Chinese Noodles, 1 c	4
Horsey Sauce, 1 oz	½	Chop Suey, 1 c, any meat	3
Potato		Chow Mein, 1 c, any meat	3
Broccoli & Cheese	7½	Egg Roll, 4"	3
Deluxe	9	Fried Rice, 1 c	4
Mushroom & Cheese	7	Moo Goo Gai Pan	6
Taco	8½	Rice, 1 c	3
Potato cakes, 2	2½		
Roast Beef		**BRAUM'S**	
Deluxe	6½	Hamburger	6
Junior	3	Cheeseburger	5
Regular	4½	Steak Sandwich	8½
Super	8½	French Fries	
Roasted Chicken	3½	Large order	5
Shake		Small order	2½
**Chocolate, small	5	**Ice Cream Cone, one dip	2½
**Jamocha, small	5½		
**Vanilla, small	4½		

*75 calories = 1 point
**Contains too much sugar

219

Menu Items	Calorie Points*	Menu Items	Calorie Points*
BURGER KING		**Ice Cream Cone, small	2
Bacon Double Cheeseburger	8	**Ice Cream Cone, regular	3
Cheeseburger	5	**Ice Cream Cone, large	4½
Double	7	Dilly Bar	3
French Fries, regular	3	Fish Sandwich	5½
Hamburger	4	with Cheese	6
Double	5½	French Fries	
Onion Rings, regular	3½	Regular	3½
Specialty Chicken		Large	4½
Sandwich	7½	Hamburger	5
Specialty Ham & Cheese		Double	7
Sandwich	7½	Triple	9½
Whaler Sandwich	7½	Hot Dog	4
with Cheese	8	Hot Dog with Cheese	4½
Whopper Jr.	5	Hot Dog with Chili	4½
with Cheese	5½	Onion Rings, regular	4
Whopper	9	Super Hot Dog	7
Double	12	with Cheese	8
Whopper with Cheese	10	with Chili	8
Double	13		
Veal Parmigiana	8	**DENNY'S**	
		Beef-Adelphia	11½
Breakfast		Chicken Fried Steak	8
Croissanwich		Chicken Salad Plate	6½
Plain	3	Combo (Hamburger, Fries,	
and Bacon	7	and Salad or Soup)	12
and Sausage	8½	Fried Chicken	13
with Cheese	4½	Low-Calorie Plate	6
with Egg	4½		
with Egg & Cheese	6	**GODFATHER'S PIZZA**	
		Pizza, ½ of small (10") pizza	
CHURCH'S FRIED CHICKEN		Beef	7
		Combination	9½
1 Piece Chicken	4	Ham & Cheese Sandwich	7½
2 Large Pieces with		Pepperoni	7½
Dinner Roll	9	Sausage	8
3 Large Pieces with		Supreme Sandwich	9
Dinner Roll	13		
Coleslaw	1	**GRANDY'S**	
Corn on the Cob	2	Baked Beans	2
Dinner Roll	1	BBQ Ribs	
French Fries	3½	Coleslaw or Beans,	
Fried Okra	3	BBQ Sauce, Roll and 2 Ribs	11
		and 3 Ribs	14
DAIRY QUEEN		Coleslaw	1
Cheeseburger	5½	Country Fried Steak, Gravy,	
Double	9	Potatoes, Coleslaw or Beans,	
Triple	11	and 2 Rolls	9½
Chicken Sandwich	9	French Fries	4

*75 calories = 1 point
**Contains too much sugar

Menu Items	Calorie Points*
Fried Chicken	
1 Piece, Vegetable, and Roll	5
2 Pieces of Chicken, Coleslaw or Beans, and Roll	8½
Hot Biscuit Sandwich	4
with Bacon	4
with Egg & Cheese	6
with Sausage	6
Hotcakes	
with Bacon	4
with Breakfast Steak	8
with Sausage	6
One Biscuit and Gravy	4
Scrambled Eggs	
with Bacon	9½
with Breakfast Steak	13½
with Hash Browns, Biscuit, Gravy	
with Sausage	12
**"Sinnamon" roll	5
**Syrup, 1 tbsp	1

GRINDER MAN

Menu Items	Calorie Points*
Mini: Coppocollo, Black or Red	8½
Mini: Grinder	7
Mini: Hero	7½
Mini: Meatball, Club, Turkey, Pepperoni & Provolone, or Pepperoni & Mozzarella	5½
Mini: Pastrami	6½
Mini: Peppered Beef, Roast Beef, Canadian Bacon, Italian Style Ham, Sausage, or Ham	6
Mini: Reuben, Mozzarella & Sauce, or Ham/Rye	4½
Mini: Sicilian Red or Genoa	8
Mini: Vegetarian, or Provolone & Sauce	5

HARDEE's

Breakfast

Menu Items	Calorie Points*
Bacon & Egg	5½
Biscuit	3½
Fried Egg	1½
Gravy	5½
Ham	4½
Ham & Egg	6
Hash Rounds	1½
Sausage	5½

*75 calories = 1 point
**Contains too much sugar

Menu Items	Calorie Points*
Sausage & Egg	7
Steak	5½
Steak & Egg	7

Other Items

Menu Items	Calorie Points*
**Apple Turnover	4
Bacon Cheeseburger	9½
**Big Cookie	4
Big Deluxe	7½
Big Roast Beef	5½
Cheeseburger	4½
Chef Salad	3½
Chicken Fillet	7
Fisherman's Fillet	6½
French Fries, small	3
French Fries, large	5
Hamburger	4
Hot Dog	4½
Hot Ham 'n' Cheese	5
Mushroom 'n' Swiss	7
Roast Beef Sandwich	5
Shrimp Salad	5
Turkey club	6

KFC
(Kentucky Fried Chicken)

Menu Items	Calorie Points*
Chicken Breast Sandwich	6
Coleslaw, ½ c	1½
Corn, 5½" ear	2½
Extra-Crispy Chicken	
Drumstick	2
Keel	4
Side Breast	4
Thigh	4½
Wing	2½
Extra-Crispy Dinner (includes Mashed Potatoes, Gravy, Coleslaw Roll), and Drumstick & Thigh	10½
Wing & Side Breast	10
Wing & Thigh	12
Gravy, 1 tbsp	½
Kentucky Fries (3.4 oz)	2½
Mashed Potatoes (3 oz)	1
Original Recipe Chicken	
Drumstick	1½
Keel	3
Side Breast	2½
Thigh	3½
Wing	2
Original Recipe Dinner (includes Mashed Potatoes, Gravy, Coleslaw, Roll), and Drumstick & Thigh	8½

Menu Items	Calorie Points*
Wing & Side Breast	8
Wing & Thigh	9
Roll	1

LONG JOHN SILVER'S SEAFOOD SHOPPE

Menu Items	Calorie Points*
Chicken Planks	6
Clam Dinner (6 oz Clams, 3 oz Fries, 4 oz Coleslaw)	12
Coleslaw, 4 oz	2
Corn on the Cob, 1 ear	2½
Fish, 1 piece	2½
Fish, 2 pieces	5
Fish, 3 pieces	7½
Fish & Chicken Dinner (1 Fish, 2 Chicken Planks, 3 oz Fries, 4 oz Coleslaw)	11½
Fish & Fries (3 Fish, 3 oz Fries)	11½
Fish & More (2 Fish, 2 Hush Puppies, 3 oz Fries, 4 oz Coleslaw)	12
French Fries (3 oz)	4
Hush Puppies	1½
Oyster Dinner (6 Oysters, 3 oz Fries, 4 oz Coleslaw)	11
Peg Legs, 5	6
Scallop Dinner (6 Scallops, 3 oz Fries, 4 oz Coleslaw)	9½
Seafood Platter (1 Fish, 2 Scallops, 2 Shrimp, 2 Hush Puppies, 3 oz Fries, 4 oz Coleslaw)	12
Shrimp, 6 pieces	3½
Treasure Chest (2 Fish, 2 Peg Legs, 3 oz Fries, 4 oz Coleslaw)	13

LONGNECKER'S

Menu Items	Calorie Points*
Hamburger II	6
"The Hamburger"	8
Fries	5
Hot Dog, plain	7
Steak Sandwich	7

McDONALD'S

Breakfast

Menu Items	Calorie Points*
Biscuits	
Bacon, Egg & Cheese	6½
Biscuit only	4½
Sausage	6½
Sausage & Egg	8
English Muffin with Butter	2½
Hash Brown Potatoes (½ c)	1½

Menu Items	Calorie Points*
McMuffins	
Egg	4½
Sausage	6
Sausage with Eggs	7
Scrambled Eggs	2½

Other Items

Menu Items	Calorie Points*
**Apple Pie	3½
Big Mac	7½
Cheeseburger	4½
Chicken McNuggets, 6 pieces	4½
**BBQ Sauce	1
**Honey Sauce	½
Hot Mustard Sauce	1
** Sweet-Sour Sauce	1
**Chocolate-Chip Cookies	4½
**Ice Cream Cone	2½
Filet-o-Fish	6
French Fries, regular	3
Hamburger	3½
McD.L.T.	8
**McDonaldland Cookies	4
McPizza	4½
Quarter Pounder	6
with Cheese	7

PIZZA HUT***

Menu Items	Calorie Points*
Calizza	
5-Cheese, whole	8½
Italian Sausage, whole	9
Pan Pizza (2 slices)	
Cheese	8½
Pepperoni	9
Supreme	9½
Super Supreme	9
Personal Pan Pizza	
Pepperoni, whole	8
Supreme, whole	9
Priazzo Italian Pie (2 slices)	
Roma	8
Milano	7½
Thin & Crispy Pizza (2 slices)	
Cheese	6
Pepperoni	6½
Supreme	8½
Super Supreme	8

*75 calories = 1 point
**Contains too much sugar
***Based on medium, 10" pizza

Menu Items	Calorie Points*	Menu Items	Calorie Points*
RAX		Roast Sandwich	
Barbeque Beef Sandwich	4½	Scallops, steamed (3½ oz)	1
Beef, Bacon & Cheddar Sandwich	9	Shore Platter	11
Big Rax Roast Beef	7½	Shrimp, boiled (3½ oz)	1
Chicken Noodle Soup	2	Sirloin Steak (3½ oz)	4½
Chicken Sandwich	8	Snapper	1½
Chocolate-Chip Cookie	2	Snow Crab, boiled (3½ oz)	1
Chowder	2½	Sole (3½ oz)	1
French Fries	4½	Steak & Lobster Dinner	21
Ham 'n' Cheese Sandwich	4½	Tuna (3½ oz)	1½
Philly Beef 'n' Cheese Sandwich	7	Turbot (3½ oz)	1
Baked Potato		Whiting (3½ oz)	1½
Bacon & Cheese	8		
Beef Barbecue	9½	**SCHLOTSKY'S**	
Beef Stroganoff	7½	Original, small	4
Broccoli & Cheese	7½	Original, medium	8
Margarine	5½	Original, large	16
Mexican	8	Roast Sandwich	
Pizza	6½	Medium	4½
Plain	3½	Large	5½
Sour Cream	4½	Turkey Sandwich, medium	4
Potato Skins		Turkey Sandwich, large	5
Bacon & Cheese Single	1½	**SONIC**	
Rax Roast Beef	6	Hamburger	6
Turkey Bacon Club Sandwich	7½	Cheeseburger	7½
Vegetable Soup	1	Steak Sandwich	8½
		Fish Sandwich	5½
RED LOBSTER		Corn Dog	6
(Fish baked unless otherwise noted)		Coney	7½
Albacore Tuna (3½ oz)	2	Chili Pie	6½
Breaded Fried Pollock (3½ oz)	2½	French Fries	4
Breaded Fried Whiting (3½ oz)	2½	Onion Rings	5
Broiled Fisherman's Platter	13	**Twist on Cone	4
Broiled Stuffed Flounder Dinner	14		
Clams (3½ oz)	1	**SPANGLES**	
Flounder (3½ oz)	1	**Apple Pie	6
Freshwater Catfish	1½	BBQ Chicken Sandwich	7
Fried Chicken, 4 pieces	6	BBQ Ham Sandwich	4
Garlic Bread, 1 slice	2	BLT Burger (½ lb)	7
Grouper (3½ oz)	1	Chicken Club	14
Haddock (3½ oz)	1	Chicken Sandwich	13
Halibut (3½ oz)	1	Chili Dog	9
Hamburger (3 oz)	3½	Chili Frito Dish	13
Hush Puppies (2)	2½	Chili with Beans	
Lobster (3½ oz)	1½	Small	3½
Mariner's Platter	13	Large	7
Oysters (3½ oz)	1	Corn Dog	4½
Perch (3½ oz)	1	Corn Dog with Cheese	5
Pollock (3½ oz)	1	French Fries, small	3
Potato	1	French Fries, large	5
Sample Platter	11	Hamburger	5½
		Triple	11½

Menu Items	Calorie Points*
Hickory Bacon	
Burger (¼ lb)	6½
Double (½ lb)	9½
Hot Dog	9
Kraut Dog	8½
Onion Rings	9
Polish Sausage	9½
Potato	
Bacon & Cheese	7½
BBQ Beef & Cheese	9½
Broccoli & Cheese	7½
Cheese	8
Chili & Cheese	8½
Sour Cream & Chives	7
Shredded Ham Sandwich	4

STEAK AND ALE

French Onion Soup	3½

Dinner Entrees

Alaskan King Crab Feast	5
Beef & Shrimp Kabob	5
Broiled Shrimp Pilaf with Rice	6
Hawaiian Chicken (one breast) with Rice	5½
Kensington Club	8
Lobster Catch	4
Drawn Butter (1 tbsp)	1½
Petit Filet, trimmed (6 oz)	4½
Prime Rib, trimmed (8 oz)	6
Stuffed Flounder Maitre d'	6

***SUB AND STUFF

Ham & Cheese	5½
Roast Beef	5
Sub & Stuff	6½
Sub Special	5½
Tuna	7
Turkey	5

TACO BELL

Bean Burrito	4½
Beef Burrito	6½
Beefy Tostada	4
Bellbeefer	3
Bellbeefer with Cheese	4
Burrito Supreme	6

*75 calories = 1 point
**Contains too much sugar
***6-inch sandwiches made with onion, lettuce, tomato, green pepper, and black olives on white or wheat bread

Menu Items	Calorie Points*
Combination Burrito	5½
Enchilada	4
Enchirito	6
Taco	2½
Taco Burger	2½
Taco Dinner (Taco, Beans, Enchilada, Chips)	9½
Taco Salad	7½
Taco Supreme	3½
Tostado, regular	2½
Refried Beans	3
Sancho	5
Soft Taco	2½

VILLAGE INN

Breakfast

Bacon	2
Egg, one	1½
Eggs Benedict: Toasted English Muffin Topped with Canadian-style Bacon, 2 Poached Eggs, and Hollandaise with Hash Browns	10
Eggs, two	2½
English Muffin	3
French Toast	7½
Ham	3
Hash Browns	3
Omelettes	
Cheese	7
Ham & Cheese	8
Three Egg	4½
Western	6
Pancakes, three	3
Robert E. Lee: Buttermilk Biscuits, Country Gravy, and Hash Browns	10
Sausage	6
Toast	3

WENDY'S

Breakfast

Bacon, 2 strips	1½
Breakfast Sandwich	5
**Danish, 1 piece	5
French Toast, 2 slices	5½
Home Fries	5
Omelettes	
Ham & Cheese	3½
Ham, Cheese & Mushroom	4
Ham, Cheese, Onion, & Green Pepper	4
Mushroom, Onion, & Green Pepper	3

Menu Items	Calorie Points*	Menu Items	Calorie Points*
Sausage, 1 pattie	2½	French Fries	3
Scrambled Eggs	2½	Hamburger	2
Toast with Margarine, 2 slices	3½		

YOGURT HEAVEN

Other Items		**Frozen Yogurt (4 oz)	2
Cheeseburger	6½	**Tofree (4 oz)	1½
Double	9		

SALAD BAR INGREDIENTS

Chicken Sandwich	4½	††Bean Sprouts, ⅓ c	0
Chili (8 oz)	3½	††Beets, ½ c	0
French Fries, regular	4	††Bell Pepper (¼ c)	0
**Frosty Dairy Dessert (12 oz)	5½	††Cabbage, Red, ½ c	0
Hamburger	5	††Carrot, ½	0
Double	8	††Cauliflower, ½ c	0
Hot Stuffed Baked Potato (plain)	3½	Cheese, American, 2 tbsp	1½
Bacon & Cheese	7½	Coleslaw, ½ c	1
Broccoli & Cheese	7	Cottage Cheese, ⅓ c	1
Cheese	8	Croutons, ½ c	1
Chicken à la King	4½	††Cucumber, 4 slices	0
Sour Cream & Chives	6	Eggs, chopped, ½ c	1
Stroganoff & Sour Cream	6½	Kidney Beans, ⅓ c	1
Pasta Salad (½ c)	2	††Lettuce, chopped, 2 c	0
Side Salad	1½	††Mushrooms, fresh, ½ c	0
Taco Salad	5½	Potato Salad, ½ c	2½
		††Radishes, ½ c	0
Salad Bar		Raisins, 2 tbsp	½
Breadstick	½	††Red Onions, ½ c	0
Cheese, Imitation (1 oz)		††Spring Onions, 2 medium	0
American	1	Sunflower Seeds, 1 tbsp	1
Cheddar	1	††Tomatoes, Cherry, 3 medium	0
Mozzarella	1		
Swiss	1	**Salad Dressing (1 tbsp)**	
Dressings (½ tbsp)		Blue Cheese	1
Blue Cheese	1	Celery Seed	1
Celery Seed	1	Golden Italian	1
Golden Italian	1	Ranch	1
Ranch	1	Red French	1
Red French	1	Thousand Island	1
Thousand Island	1		
Reduced-Calorie Dressing (1 tbsp)		**Reduced-Calorie Dressing (1 tbsp)**	
Bacon & Tomato	½	Bacon & Tomato	½
Creamy Cucumber	½	Creamy Cucumber	½
Italian	½	Italian	½
Sunflower Seeds & Raisins (¼ c)	2½	Thousand Island	½
		Wine Vinegar	0

WHITE CASTLE

Cheeseburger	2½	**Soft Drinks (12 oz)**	
Fish Sandwich	2½	**Coca-Cola	2
		**Diet Coke	0
		**Orange Drink	2
		**Pepsi Cola	2
*75 calories = 1 point		**Diet Pepsi	0
**Contains too much sugar		**Root Beer	2
††Choice of any three = ½ calorie point		**Sprite	2

Appendix F

Metabolic (MET) Levels of Activities

Definitions

MET—The metabolic rate refers to oxygen consumption. (Note: Values do not refer to duration of effort or total expenditure over some period of time.)

Static Tension (+)—Static, or isometric, component of an activity that increases the work required of the heart.

Points to consider before initiating specific tasks:

1. MET level at which you are functioning.
2. Environment: temperature, clothing, emotional stress, position.
3. Duration: You should have full recovery without fatigue within an hour of activity.

Calculation of METs:
Duration of activity (in hours or portions of hours) × MET number = subtotal of METs. Sum of subtotal of METs = total METs. (Average adult is expected to accumulate 30 to 40 METs per day.)

ACTIVITIES LISTED BY MET LEVELS

SELF-CARE METS

Sitting in a chair	1.0
Care for fingernails	1.2
Brush teeth	1.2
Eating a meal	1.3
Wash hands and face	1.5
Wash upper body	1.5
Bathe in tub	1.5
Comb hair, male and female	1.5
Sit on edge of bed	1.5
Sit on bedside commode	1.5
Wash hair, male and female	1.5+
Shave, electric and safety razor	1.6
Set hair	1.6+
Wash entire body sitting in bathroom	1.7+
Shower, sit	1.8+
Dress and undress nightclothes	2.0+
street clothes	2.0+
Shower, stand	3.8
Use bedpan	4.8

HOUSEWORK

Machine sewing, household	2.3
Wash clothes (by machine)	2.3+
Washing small clothes	2.5
Mix batter	2.5+
Fix simple meal (breakfast or lunch)	2–3.0
Fold clothes	2–3.0+
Making bed	2–3.0++
Fix complex meal (dinner)	3.0+
Wash dishes	3.0+
Ironing, standing	3.0++
Scrubbing at counter height, standing	3.0++
Bending and stooping (picking up newspaper)	3.0++
Peel potatoes	3.2
Cleaning stove (inside)	3–4.0++
Scrub pots and pans	3–4.0++
Dusting/polishing (reaching with arms)	3–4.0++
Changing bed	3–4.0++
Mopping floors (hand and knees)	3–5.0++
Vacuuming (bare floor to pile rugs)	3–5.0++
Sweeping floor	4–5.0++
Mopping (standing)	4–5.0++
Grocery shopping	4–5.0++++
Scrubbing, polishing, waxing floors, walls, cars, windows, while standing	5–6.0+++
Turning mattress	7.0+++++

VOCATIONAL

Sitting at desk, writing, calculating	1.5
Lying under a car to repair	1.5
Using hand tools	1.8
Light assembly work	1.8
Radio repair	1.8
Driving a truck	1.8
Working heavy levers	2.0
Dredge	2.0
Watch repairing	2.1
Bookbinding, light	2.3
Typing rapidly	2.3
Power sanding or sawing	2.6
Armature winding	2.6
Bricklaying	3–5.0+++
Plastering	3–5.0+++
Pushing wheelbarrow, 50 lb	4.0++++
Wringing by hand	4.5
Hanging wash	4.6
Carpentry Lift maximum 50 lb;	4–6.0++++
frequently lift/carry 25 lb	4–6.0++++
Shoveling	5–7.0++++
Digging holes	5–7.0++++
Chopping wood	5–7.0++++
Light/heavy farming	5–7.0+++
Light/heavy industrial	5–7.0+++
Lift maximum 100 lb; frequently lift/carry 50 lb	6–8.0+++++

AVOCATIONAL/RECREATIONAL

Phoning, conversation	1.0
Leather punching, lacing, back supported	1.8
Leather tooling, back supported	1.8
Making link belt, back supported	1.9
Rug hooking, sitting	1.9
Hand sewing	2.0

Knitting, 23 stitches/min	2.0	Sexual activity	3–5.0+++
Embroidery	2.0	Canoeing, 2–5 mph	3–6.0+++
Playing cards or any		Spading	3–8.0
sitting competitive game	2.0	Playing drums	4.3
Chip carving, back supported	2.1	Bowling	4.5
Copper tooling	2.2	Badminton	4.5
Weaving, table loom	2.2	Walking down stairs	4.5
Leather carving, sitting	2.3	Gardening	4.7
Painting, sitting	2.5	Ping-Pong	4–5.0
Chisel carving with mallet, sitting	2.5	Archery	4–5.0
Printing (hand composition)	2.6	Hunting	4–6.0
Playing piano	2–3.0++	Hoeing	4–6.0++
Sailing	2–5.0+	Golfing	4–7.0
Horseshoes	3.0	Swimming, breaststroke,	
Walking, 2.5 mph	3.0+	20 yd/min	5.0
Hammering	3.0+++	Walking, 3.5 mph	5.5+
Horseback riding, walk	3.3	Sawing wood	5–7.0
Playing organ, sitting	3.5	Ice skating	5–7.0
Lift 20 lb maximum;		Dancing, fox-trot	5–7.0+++
frequently lift 10 lb	3.5+++	Tennis	5–15.0+
Volleyball	3.8	Horseback riding, trotting	7.5
Planting	3–4.0	Cycling, 13 mph	7–9.0
Riding motorcycle	3–4.0+++	Mowing lawn by hand or power	8.0
Painting wall	3–4.0++	Skiing (snow or water)	9.0
Cycling, 5.5 mph	3–4.0+++	Squash	9.0
Weeding	3–5.0+		

Appendix G

Some Activity and Exercise Caloric Expenditures

The following are lists of various activities and classifications of work and recreation in relation to calories expended per minute.

Activity	Calories Per Minute	Activity	Calories Per Minute
Work		Conversing	1.4
Rest	1.25	Dressing, undressing	2.3
Light	2.5	Washing hands, face, brushing hair	2.5
Moderate	5.0	Washing and dressing	2.6
Heavy	7.5	Washing and shaving	2.6
Very heavy	10.0	Using bedside commode	3.6
Extremely heavy	12.5	Showering	4.2
		Using a bedpan	4.7
Locomotion			
Wheelchair, 1.2 mph	2.4	**Household Tasks**	
Walking, 2.5 mph	3.6	Hand sewing	1.4
Walking down stairs	5.2	Knitting	1.5
Walking, 2.75 mph	5.6	Ironing, standing	1.7
Walking with crutches	8.0	Simple work, sitting	1.7
and/or braces, 1.2 mph		Machine sewing	1.8
Walking up stairs		Peeling potatoes	2.0
(17-lb load, 27 ft/min)	9.0	Brushing boots	2.2
Walking up stairs (no load)	8.0	Polishing	2.4
		Scrubbing, standing	2.9
Exercises		Washing small clothes	3.0
Bending at waist (sideways),		Bringing in wash	3.3
13/min	2.2	Kneading dough	3.3
Sitting on floor, touching toes		Scrubbing floors	3.6
15/min	2.4	Cleaning windows	3.7
Balancing exercises	2.5	Making beds	3.9
Abdominal exercises	3.0	Mopping	4.2
Lying on floor, leg raising, 10/min	3.5	Wringing by hand	4.4
Arm swinging, hopping	6.5	Hanging wash	4.5
Push-ups, 16/min	7.5	Polishing floors	4.8
		Beating carpets	4.9
Self-care		Breaking firewood	4.9
Resting, supine	1.0	Stripping and making bed	5.4
Sitting	1.2	Cleaning floors, kneeling, bending	6.0
Standing, relaxed	1.4		
Eating	1.4		

231

Activity	Calories Per Minute	Activity	Calories Per Minute
Children's Recreation		Mechanical typewriter, 30 w/min	1.39
Sitting, listening to radio	1.0	Mechanical typewriter, 40 w/min	1.48
Sitting, playing with puzzle	1.2	Misc. office work, sitting	1.6
Sitting, singing	1.4	Misc. office work, standing	1.8
Standing, drawing	1.5–1.9	***Light Engineering Work***	
		Watch and clock repair	1.6
Recreation		Light assembly line	1.8
Sitting, writing	1.9–2.2	Draftsman	1.8
Painting	2.0	Armature winding	2.2
Sitting, listening to radio	2.0–2.5	Light machine work	2.4
Playing cards	2.2	Radio assembly	2.7
Cycling	2.4–3.1	***Printing Industry***	
Playing piano	2.5	Hand composition	2.2
Playing violin	2.7	Printing	2.2
Driving car	2.8	Paper laying	2.5
Canoeing, 2.5 mph	3.0	***Press Goods Industry***	
Horseback riding, slow	3.0	Pressing household utensils	3.8
Playing volleyball	3.5	Carpentry	3.0
Playing with children	3.5	***Locksmith***	
Playing drums	4.0–4.2	Five other processes	2.1–2.9
Sculling, 51 m/min, 12 mph	4.1	Filing with large file	3.3–3.7
Bowling	4.4	***Tailor***	
Cycling, 5.5 mph	4.5	Hand sewing	2.0–2.9
Golf	5.0	Cutting	2.4–2.7
Archery	5.2	Machine sewing	2.8–2.9
Dancing	5.5	Pressing	3.5–4.3
Gardening, weeding	5.6	Ironing	4.2
Recreational swimming	6–7.0	***Leather Trade***	
Tennis	7.1	Polishing shoes	1.8
Horseback riding, at a trot	8.0	Filing soles	2.3
Spading	8.6	Fixing soles	2.4
Gardening, digging	8.6	Shoe repairing	2.7
Playing football	8.9	Shoe manufacturing	3.0
Skiing	9.9	***Mail Carrier***	
Swimming, breaststroke, 40 yd/min	10.0	Climbing stairs	8.0
Playing soccer	10.2	Postal load, 24.2 lb (11 kg)	9.8
Climbing slope	10.7	Postal load, 35.2 lb (16 kg)	9.8–13.8
Cycling, 13 mph	11.0	***Pick, Shovel, and Wheelbarrow***	
Swimming, sidestroke, 20 yd/min	11.0	Wheelbarrow, 115 lb (52 kg)	5.0
Swimming, backstroke, 40 yd/min	11.5	Hoeing with pick	7.0
Swimming, crawl, 45 yd/min	11.5	Shoveling, 17.6 lb (8 kg) load, 12 throws/min, 1 meter lift	7.5
		Shoveling, 16 lb (7 kg)	8.5
Occupations		Shoveling, 17.6 lb (8 kg) load, 12 throws/min, 2 meter lift	9.5
Clerical Work		***Building Industry***	
Electric typewriter, 30 w/min	1.16	Measuring wood	2.4
Electric typewriter, 40 w/min	1.31	Machine sawing	2.4

Activity	Calories Per Minute	Activity	Calories Per Minute
Light work laying stones or bricks	3.4	Using heavy hammer	6.3–9.8
Measuring and sawing	3.5	Drilling hardwood	7.0
Misc. work, carrying	3.6	Planing hardwood	9.1
Shaping stones with mason's hammer	3.8	***Miscellaneous***	
Making wall with bricks and mortar	4.0	Tractor	4.2
		Plowing	5.9
Plastering	4.1	Haying	7.3
Joining floor boards	4.4	Mowing lawn by hand	7.3
Mixing cement	4.7	Felling a tree	8.0
Chiseling	5.7	Tending a furnace	10.2
Sawing softwood	6.3	Climbing a hill or set of stairs with a 22-lb (10-kg) load, 54 ft/min	16.2
Sawing hardwood	6.3		

Appendix H

Resources

Abbott Laboratories
MediSense Products
4A Crosby Drive
Bedford, MA 01730
800-527-3339

Activa Brand Products, Inc.
36 Fourth Street
Charlottetown, PE
Canada C1E 2B3
800-011-6771

**American Association of
Diabetes Educators**
100 West Monroe
Chicago, IL 60623
800-338-DMED
Fax 312-661-1700
*Educational material and information about
diabetes educators*

American Diabetes Association
1660 Duke Street
Alexandria, VA 22314
800-232-3472
*Educational material, research programs,
and association information*

American Foundation for the Blind
11 Penn Plaza, Suite 300
New York, NY 10001
800-232-5463
*Catalog, supplies, and information
for the blind*

**American Medical
Systems, Inc.**
10700 Bren Road West
Minnetonka, MN 55343
612-933-4666

American Vision and Diagnostics, Inc.
1301 West 22nd Street
Suite 312
Oakbrook, IL 60521
630-368-7510

Animas Corporation
590 Lancaster Avenue
Frazer, PA 19355
877-YES-PUMP
Insulin infusion pump

Aventis Pharmaceuticals
399 Interpace Parkway
Parsippany, NJ 07054
800-981-2491, Ext. 6000
Oral agent, designer insulin

Ascensia
Customer Service Department
Bayer Corporation
Diagnostic Division
P.O. Box 2020
Mishawaka, IN 46546-9913
800-348-8100
Education materials and meters

BD (Becton Dickinson Consumer Products)
One Becton Drive
Franklin Lakes, NJ 07417-1883
800-237-4554
*Educational material and
product information, syringes*

Bioject, Inc.
7620 SW Bridgeport Road
Portland, OR 97224
800-848-2538
Insulin injector

Bristol-Myers Squibb
1350 Liberty Avenue
Hillside, NJ 07207
800-468-7746

Canadian Diabetes Association
15 Toronto Street, Suite 800
Toronto, ON
Canada M5C 2E3
416-363-3373

Can-Am Care Corporation
200 Prospect Street
Waltham, MA 02453
800-899-7353
*Lancets, glucose tabs, blood glucose
test strips*

Cell Robotics Inc.
2715 Broadbent Parkway
Albuquerque, NM 87107
800-846-0590
Lasette

C.R. Bard, Inc.
Urological Division
Covington, GA 30209
ESKA Jonas Silicon-Silver penile prosthesis

Diabetes Supplies, Inc.
275 Curry Hollow Road
Pittsburgh, PA 15236
412-650-9734

Disetronic Medical Systems, Inc.
5151 Program Avenue
St. Paul, MN 55112
800-280-7801
Insulin infusion pump

Eli Lilly and Company
Consumer Relations
Lilly Corp. Center
Indianapolis, IN 46285
800-545-5979
*Educational material and
product information*

Equidyne Systems, Inc.
11770 Bernardo Plaza Court, Suite 351
San Diego, CA 92128
877-474-6539
Insulin injector device

Health Education Associates, Inc.
8 San Sebastian Way, Unit 13
Sandwich, MA 02563
508-888-8044

HemoCue, Inc.
23263 Madero
Mission Viejo, CA 92691
949-859-2630
Device for screening and monitoring

Home Diagnostics
2400 NW 55th Court
Fort Lauderdale, FL 33309
800-342-7226
Blood-glucose meters

Hypoguard
7301 Ohms Lane, Suite 200
Edina, MN 55439-2331
800-818-8877
Pump supplies, lancets, meter

ICN Pharmaceuticals, Inc.
3300 Hayland Avenue
Costa Mesa, CA 92626
800-548-5100
Diabetes medications, instaglucose

Identi-Find
P.O. Box 567
Canton, NC 28716
828-648-6768
Medical identification

I.D. Technology, Inc.
117 Nelson Road
Baltimore, MD 23208-1111
877-IDBANDS

Independent Living Aids, Inc.
27 East Mall
Plainview, NY 11803
516-752-8080
Supplies

Insuleeve
P.O. Box 453
Fair Lawn, NJ 07410
201-796-3170
Injection assist device

International Diabetes Federation
40 Washington Street
Brussels, Belgium 1050

Juvenile Diabetes Foundation
120 Wall Street
New York, NY 10005
800-223-1138
Educational material and information

Lifescan Inc.
1000 Gibraltar
Milpitas, CA 95035
800-227-8862
Blood-glucose meter

Lighthouse Catalog
111 East 59th Street
New York, NY 10022
800-829-0500
Products for the visually impaired

Medical Alert Foundation International
2323 Colorado Avenue
Turlock, CA 95381
800-432-5378
Medical identification

Medicool, Inc.
23520 Telo Avenue
Suite #6
Torrance, CA 90575
800-433-2469
Injectors

Medi-Ject Corporation
161 Cheshire Lane, Suite 100
Minneapolis, MN 55441
800-328-3074
Needle-free injectors

Mentor Corporation
5425 Hollister Avenue
Santa Barbara, CA 93111
805-681-6000
Mentor GFS penile prosthesis, Mentor penile prosthesis, Small-Carrion prosthesis

Metrika, Inc.
510 Oakmead Parkway
Sunnyvale, CA 94085
877-A1C-4-YOU
Portable A1c meter

MiniMed, Inc.
18000 West Devonshire Road
Northridge, CA 91325
800-933-3322
Insulin infusion pump

National Diabetes Information Clearinghouse (NDIC)
Bethesda, MD 20892-3560
301-654-3327
Education Information

National Emergency Medicine Association (NEMA)
306 West Joppa Road
Towson, MD 21204
800-332-6362 (except MD)
301-494-0300 (MD only)
Daytime hours and recorded answering device; information

Novo-Nordisk Pharmaceuticals, Inc.
100 Overlook Center
Suite 200
Princeton, NJ 08540
800-727-6500
Educational material, product information, insulins

Ortho-McNeil Pharmaceuticals, Inc.
1000 Route 202
P.O. Box 300
Raritan, NJ 08869-0802
888-734-7263
Wound care treatment

Osbon Medical Systems
P.O. Box 1478
Augusta, GA 30903-1478
800-438-8592 or
612-858-9311
DuraPhaw prosthesis, OmniPhase prosthesis, Snap-Gauge, EricAid System

Paddock Laboratories
3940 Quebec Avenue North
Minneapolis, MN 55427
800-328-5113

Palco Laboratories
8030 Soquel Avenue, Suite 104
Santa Cruz, CA 95062
800-346-4488
Injectors

Parke-Davis
201 Tabor Road
Morris Plains, NJ 07950
888-900-TYPE2
800-223-0432
Fax 973-540-2000
Blood pressure medicine

Pharmacia + Upjohn Company
95 Corporate Drive
P.O. Box 6995
Bridgewater, NJ 08807
908-901-8000
Oral agents

Resources for Rehabilitation
33 Bedford Street, Suite 19A
Lexington, MA 02173
617-862-6455

Revive System Corporation
Box 592
Lake Geneva, WI 53147
414-248-2590
Revive System for sexual dysfunction

Roche Diagnostics
(formerly Boehringer Mannheim)
9115 Hague Road
P.O. Box 50100
Indianapolis, IN 46250-0100
800-858-8072
Blood-glucose meters, educational materials, product information

SmithKline Beecham Pharmaceuticals
One Franklin Plaza
P.O. Box 7929
Philadelphia, PA 19101
800-366-8900, Ext. 5231
Oral agents

Surgitek Medical Engineering Corp.
3037 Mount Pleasant Street
Racine, WI 53404
414-639-7205
Flexi-flate prosthesis, Flexi-rod prosthesis, Uni-Flate 1000

Takeda Pharmaceuticals America, Inc.
Millbrook Business Center
475 Half Day Road, Suite 500
Lincolnshire, IL 60069

University of Michigan
Media Union Library
3281 Bonisteel Boulevard
Ann Arbor, MI 48109-2094
Educational materials

Vitajet Precision Instruments, Inc.
Mada Equipment Co., Inc.
27071 Cabot Road, Suite 110
Laguna Hills, CA 92653
800-848-2538
Jet injectors

Wal-Mart Stores, Inc.
Corporate Offices
702 SW 8th Street
Bentonville, AR 72715-8071
800-461-7448
Generic oral agents; insulins

Whittier Medical, Inc.
865 Turnpike Street
North Andover, MA 01845
800-645-1115
Supplies

For more details on products, look for the yearly published *Resource Guide of the American Diabetes Association, Supplement to Diabetes Forecast.*

Appendix I

American Diabetes Association
Division and Area Offices

CENTRAL DIVISION
2323 North Mayfair Road
Suite 502
Wauwatosa, WI 53226
414-778-5500
Jim Woods, Vice President

Central Indiana Area Office
317-352-9226

Central Ohio Area Office
614-436-1917

Cleveland Metro Area Office
440-717-1627

Gateway Area Office
314-822-5490

Greater Illinois Area Office
217-875-9011

Northeast Ohio Area Office
330-835-3149

Southeast Ohio/
Northern Kentucky Area Office
513-759-9330

Western Pennsylvania Area Office
412-824-1181

West Virginia/Southeast Ohio Area Office
304-768-2596

NORTH CENTRAL DIVISION
2323 North Mayfair Road
Suite 502
Wauwatosa, WI 53226
414-778-5500
Lew Bartfield, Vice President

Greater Michigan Area Office
616-458-9341

Iowa Area Office
515-276-2237

Minnesota Area Office
763-593-5333

Nebraska/South Dakota Area Office
402-572-3747

North Dakota Area Office
701-746-4427

Northern Illinois Area Office
312-346-1805

Michigan/Northwest Ohio Area Office
248-433-3830

Wisconsin Area Office
414-778-5500

MOUNTAIN/PACIFIC DIVISION
2480 West 26th Avenue, Suite 120B
Denver, CO 80211
720-855-1102
Mike Van Abel, Vice President

Alaska Area Office
907-272-1424

Arizona Area Office
602-861-4731

Border Area Office
520-795-3711

Colorado/Wyoming/Montana Area Office
720-855-1102

Hawaii Area Office
808-927-5979

New Mexico Area Office
505-266-5716

Oregon/Southern Idaho Area Office
503-736-2770

Utah Area Office
801-363-3024

Washington/Northern Idaho Area Office
206-282-4616

NORTHEASTERN DIVISION
149 Madison Avenue, Room 701
New York, NY 10016
212-725-4925
Joyce, Waite, Vice President

Connecticut and
Western Massachusetts Area Office
203-639-0385

Central Pennsylvania Area Office
717-657-4310

Delaware/Eastern Shore Area Office
302-656-0030

District of Columbia Metro Area Office
202-331-8303

Eastern New England Metro Area Office
617-482-4580

Greater New York City Area Office
212-725-4925

Maryland Area Office
410-265-0075

Northern New Jersey Area Office
732-469-7979

Southeastern Pennsylvania Area Office
610-828-5003

Upstate New York/Western New England
Area Office
716-835-0274

SOUTH CENTRAL DIVISION
4425 West Airport Freeway
Suite 130
Irving, TX 75062
972-255-6900
Quin Neal, Vice President

Alamo District Area Office (South Texas)
210-829-1765

Arkansas Area Office
502-221-7444

Central Texas Area Office
512-472-9838

Kansas Area Office
316-684-6091

Kansas City Area Office
913-383-8210

Louisiana Area Office
504-889-0278

Mississippi Area Office
601-932-1118

Missouri Area Office
417-890-8400

Northeast Texas/
Northern Louisiana Area Office
972-392-1181

Oklahoma Area Office
918-492-3839

Southeastern Texas Area Office
713-977-7706

West Texas Area Office
806-794-0691

SOUTH COASTAL DIVISION
1101 North Lake Destiny Road
Suite 415
Maitland, FL 32751
407-660-1926
Nancy Carlton, Vice President

Atlanta Metro/North Georgia Area Office
404-320-7100

Central Florida Area Office
407-660-1926

Northeast Florida/East Georgia Area Office
904-730-7200

Northwest Florida/Downstate Alabama
850-478-5957

Outstate Georgia Area Office
912-353-8110

Southeast Florida Area Office
305-477-8999

Southwest Florida Area Office
813-855-5007

Upstate Alabama Area Office
205-870-5172

SOUTHERN DIVISION
Two Hanover Square
4334 Fayetteville Street Mall
Suite 1650
Raleigh, NC 27601
919-743-5400
Ed Owens, Vice President

Central North Carolina Area Office
704-373-9111

Central Western Virginia Area Office
804-225-8038

Eastern North Carolina Area Office
919-743-5400

East Tennessee Area Office
865-524-7868

Greater Hampton Roads Area Office
757-455-6335

Kentucky Area Office
502-452-6072

Middle Tennessee Area Office
615-298-3066

South Carolina Area Office
864-609-5054

West Tennessee Area Office
901-682-8232

WESTERN DIVISION
2720 Gateway Oaks Drive
Sacramento, CA 95833
916-924-3232
Mike Clinkenbeard, Vice President

Los Angeles Area Office
323-966-2890

Nevada Area Office
702-369-9995

Orange County/Los Angeles Area Office
714-662-7940

Sacramento Area Office
916-924-3232

San Diego Area Office
619-234-9897

San Francisco Area Office
510-654-4499

San Jose Area Office
408-241-1922

Appendix J

Summer Camps for Children with Diabetes

Alabama
Camp Seale Harris*#
P.O. Box 1179
Killen, AL 35645
256-757-0193

Contact: Terry Ackley
Residential camp/family sessions

Alaska
Camp Kushtaka*#
801 West Firewood Lane, No. 103
Anchorage, AK 99503
907-272-1424

Contact: Michelle Cassono
Residential camp

Arizona
Camp AZDA*#
9034 North 23rd Avenue, Suite 9-B
Phoeniz, AZ 85021
602-861-4731

Contact: Sara Watson
Residential camp

Native American Research and
Training Center*
University of Arizona
1642 East Helen Street
Tucson, AZ 85719
520-621-5075

Contact: Pandora Hughes
E-mail: ahughes@ahsc.arizona.edu

Native American Youth Wellness Camp*
Prescott, AZ
For youths with Type 2 diabetes or impaired
glucose tolerance

Residential camp

Arkansas
Camp Aldersgate*#
2000 Aldersgate Road
Little Rock, AR 72205
501-225-1444

Contact: Sarah Spencer
Residential camp

California
Bearskin Meadow Camp*
Diabetic Youth Foundation
1954 Mt. Diablo Boulevard, Suite A
Walnut Creek, CA 94596
925-937-3393

Residential camp/day camp/family session

Camp Buck
Diabetes Association of Santa Clara Valley*
1165 Lincoln Avenue, Suite 300
San Jose, CA 95125
408-287-3785 or 1-800-989-1165

Contact: Tom Smith/Desiree Gaspar
Residential camp

Camp Conrad-Chinnock#
Diabetic Youth Service, Inc.
6300 Wilshire Boulevard, Suite 100
Los Angeles, CA 90048
213-966-2980, Ext. 244

Residential camp/family session

Some camp names may have been omitted due to the restructuring process. We apologize for these omissions and will do everything possible to rectify them in future editions.
* Listed with Diabetes Camping Association (DCA).
# Listed with American Diabetes Association (ADA).
It is possible that a camp may be listed with both the DCA and the ADA.

Camp Crispi*
The Diabetes Society
1165 Lincoln Avenue, Suite 300
San Jose, CA 95125
408-287-3785 or 1-800-989-1165

Camp de los Niños*
Diabetes Association of Santa Clara Valley
1165 Lincoln Avenue, Suite 300
San Jose, CA 95125
408-287-3785

Contact: Tom Smith/Desiree Gaspar
Residential camp

Camp DJ Sequoia Lake*
Diabetes Association of Santa Clara Valley
1165 Lincoln Avenue, Suite 300
San Jose, CA 95125
408-287-3785 or 1-800-989-1165

Residential camp

Camp Fox*
Diabetes Association of Santa Clara Valley
1165 Lincoln Avenue, Suite 300
San Jose, CA 95125
408-287-3785 or 1-800-989-1165

Residential camp

Camp Surf*
Diabetes Society of Santa Clara Valley
1165 Lincoln Avenue, Suite 300
San Jose, CA 95125
408-287-3785 or 1-800-989-1165

Contact: Desiree Gaspar
Residential camp

Camp Wana-Cura*#
American Diabetes Association
10445 Old Placerville Road
Sacramento, CA 95827
916-369-0999

Contact: Lisa Murdock
Day camp

Colorado
Camp Colorado*#
American Diabetes Association
Colorado/Wyoming/Montana Area
2480 West 26th Avenue, Suite 120B
Denver, CO 80210
720-855-1102, Ext. 7019

Residential camp/bike camp/wilderness
camp/equestrian camp

Connecticut/New Hampshire
Camp Carefree*#
1-800-676-4065, Ext. 3606

Contact: Joan Clifford
Residential camp

Florida
Boggy Creek Gang Camp*
30500 Brantly Branch Road
Eutis, FL 32736
352-483-4200

Diabetes family session

Camp JADA*#
American Diabetes Association
8384 Baymeadows Road, Suite 10
Jacksonville, FL 32256
800-741-6104

Contact: Sue Glass
Day camp

Camp Koral Kids*
Coral Springs Medical Center
North Broward Hospital Center
3000 Coral Springs Drive
Coral Springs, FL 33065
954-796-3990
Fax: 954-344-3000

Contact: Christina Ring
Day camp

Florida Camp for Children and Youth with
Diabetes, Inc.#
Rosalie Bandyopadhyay
P.O. Box 14136 University Station
Gainesville, FL 32604
352-334-1323

Contact: Alsonso Avendano
Residential camp/peewee adventure
camp/cycling adventure camp/
fun sports camp/family session/elementary
bring-a-friend day in December/winter camp

Georgia
Camp Juliet*
University Hospital Diabetes Services
1350 Walton Way
Augusta, GA 30901
706-774-8473

Contact: Debra Whitley
Residential camp

Camp Little Shot*
Diabetes Treatment Center of America
777 Hemlock Street
Macon, GA 31201
912-633-1531

Contact: Brady Shore
Residential camp

Camp Pacer*
204 Tilbet Avenue
Savannah, GA 31406
912-927-9537

Contact: Donna Stembeidge
Day camp

Diabetes Day Camp
American Diabetes Association*
1 Corporate Square, Suite 127
Atlanta, GA 30329
404-320-7100

Georgia Diabetes Camps, Inc.*
P.O. Box 133049
Atlanta, GA 30333
404-617-3077

Residential camp

Hawaii
Diabetes Youth Camp*#
YMCA Camp Erdman
8501 Wilei Road
Honolulu, HI 96817
808-521-1142

Idaho
Camp Hodia*
Idaho DYP
2875 Mountain View Drive
Boise, ID 83704
208-344-0407

Residential camp

Illinois
Camp Granada
American Diabetes Association*#
2580 Federal Drive, No. 403
Decatur, IL 62526
217-875-9011 or 1-800-445-1667

Contact: Donna Scott
Residential camp

Easter Seal Camp*
1230 North Highland Avenue
Aurora, IL 60506
630-896-1961

Residential camp

Teen Adventure Camp*#
Northern Illinois, ADA
30 North Michigan Avenue, Suite 2015
Chicago, IL 60602
312-346-1805, Ext. 323

Contact: Suzanne Aspey
Residential camp

Triangle D Camp
American Diabetes Association*
30 North Michigan Avenue, No. 2015
Chicago, IL 60602
312-346-1805, Ext. 323

Contact: Suzanne Aspey
Residential camp/*day camp

Camp-Can-Do/*Camp Confidence*#
Camp Crossroads*/Camp Discovery*

University of Illinois 4-H Memorial Camp
University of Illinois
RR 2, Box 136
Monticello, IL 61856 or 888-342-2383
217-762-2741

Contact: Donna Scott
Residential camp

Indiana
Camp John Warvel*#
American Diabetes Association
7363 East 21st Street
Indianapolis, IN 46219
317-352-9226 or 1-800-228-2897

Contact: Elaine McClane
Residential camp

Camp Joslin
1850 State Street
New Albany, IN 47150
812-949-5915

Contact: Beth Ackerman
Residential camp/day camp/
outdoor adventure camp

Happy Hollow Camp for
Children with Diabetes*
Diabetes Youth Foundation of Indiana
1300 Main Street
Danville, IN 46122
765-348-1762

Contact: Sam Wentworth
Residential camp/Spring Family Camp/
Tour of Friendship Summer Bicycle Trip/
Fall Family Camp

Iowa
Camp Hertko Hollow*#
American Diabetes Association
6200 Aurora Avenue, 504 W
Des Moines, IA 50322
515-276-2237

Contact: Vivian Murray
Residential camp

Kansas
Camp Discovery*#
American Diabetes Association
837 S. Hillside Street
Wichita, KS 62708-3309
316-684-6091

Contact: Susan Sanders
Residential camp/high-adventure mountain
backpacking trip

Ka-Di-Da-Ca*#
837 Hillside Street
Wichita, KS 67208
316-684-6091

Day camp

Kentucky
Camp Hendon*#
American Diabetes Association
Wattereson City Office Park
1941 Bishop Lane, Suite 110
Louisville, KY 40218
502-452-6072

Contact: Tracy Esarey
Residential camp

Fun Quest*
American Diabetes Association
Our Lady of Bellefonte Hospital
St. Christopher Drive

Ashland, KY 41101
606-833-2958

Contact: Michelle Gillum
Children's Day event

Southern Region
3703 Taylorsville Road, Suite 118
Louisville, KY 40220
502-452-1201, Ext. 3312

Louisiana
Louisiana Lions Camp for
  Children with Diabetes*#
12090 South Harrell's Ferry Road, Suite B
Baton Rouge, LA 70816
504-292-5001

Contact: Tammy Boudreaux
Residential camp

Maine
Camp Carefree*
American Diabetes Association
10 Bangor Street, Suite F
Augusta, ME 04330
1-800-413-5854

Contact: Lesha Crews
Residential camp

Camp Sunshine*
35 Acadia Road
South Casco, ME 04077
207-655-3800

Contact: Laura Bean
Residential camp

Maryland
Camp Glyndon*#
American Diabetes Association
3120 Timanus Lane, #106
Baltimore, MD 21244
410-265-0075

Contact: Jody Kakocek
Residential camp/family weekend

Massachusetts
Camp EDI
Diabetes Youth Association of
Greater Fall River, Inc.
101 Rock Street
Fall River, MA 02722
508-672-5671

Contact: Emily Chase
Day camp

Clara Barton Camp for Girls with Diabetes*#
The Barton Center for
Diabetes Education, Inc.
68 Clara Barton Road
North Oxford, MA 01537-0356
508-987-2058

Contact: Gaylen McCann
Residential camp/family session/
coed session/girls session

Elliott P. Joslin Camps for
Children with Diabetes*#
Joslin Diabetes Center
Camp Office
One Joslin Place
Boston, MA 02215
617-732-2455

Contact: Paul Madden
e-mail: camp.joslin@joslin.harvard.edu
Residential camp—boys only sessions
Wilderness leadership camp—coed sessions
Winter camp—coed session
Weekend sessions throughout school year
Life after high school program in spring—
coed session

Michigan
Camp Midicha*#
American Diabetes Association
Bingham Center
30600 Telegraph Road, No. 2255
Bingham Farms, MI 48025
248-433-3830, Ext. 227

Contact: Patricia Foy
Residential camp/canoe and horse trips

Southeast Michigan Area*
30600 Telegraph Road, Suite 2255
Bingham, MI 48025
248-433-3830, Ext. 6701

Minnesota
Camp Needlepoint and Camp Daypoint*#
American Diabetes Association
715 Florida Avenue South, Suite 307
Minneapolis, MN 55426-1759
612-593-5333, Ext. 243

Contact: Kim Krost
Needlepoint—residential camp

Daypoint—day camp

Mississippi
Camp Hopewell*
24 County Road, #231
Oxford, MS 38655
662-234-2254

Contact: Rebecca Winsett
Residential camp

Twin Lakes Diabetes Camp*#
P.O. Box 998
Jackson, MS 39205
601-372-9594

Contact: Katherine Davis
Residential camp

Missouri
Camp Day Break*#
Southeast Missouri Hospital
1701 Lacey
Cape Girardeau, MO 63701
573-334-4822

Contact: Janet Stewart
Day camp

Camp Earth Works*#
American Diabetes Association
1944A East Sunshine
Springfield, MO 65804
417-890-8400

Contact: Renée Paulsell
Day camp; sessions in
Joplin and in Springfield

Camp EDI at Kiwanis Camp Wyman;
Camp Kids (Resident & Day Camp)*#
American Diabetes Association
2650 South Hanley Road, No. 350
St. Louis, MO 63144
314-647-2110, Ext. 15

Contact: Michelle Reynolds,
or Leslie Lake at 314-822-5496
Residential camp

Camp Hickory Hill*
P.O. Box 1942
Columbia, MO 65205

573-698-2510

Contact: Pete Bakutes
Residential camp

Camp Red-Bird*#
2650 South Hanley Road, No. 350
St. Louis, MO 63144
314-647-2110, Ext. 15

Contact: Michelle Reynolds
Residential camp

Camp Shawnee*#
American Diabetes Association
9201 Ward Parkway, No. 300
Kansas City, MO 64114
816-361-3361

Contact: Mary
Residential camp

Montana
Camp Diamont*
American Diabetes Association
P.O. Box 2411
Great Falls, MT 59403
460-761-0908 or 1-800-232-6668

Residential camp

Montana's Youth Retreat*#
460-256-0616

Contact: Mary Hernandez
Residential camp

Nebraska
Camp Cosmo*
Community Health
3700 Avenue B
Scottsbluff, NE 69361
308-630-1559

Contact: Kim Croft
Residential/day camp/family program

Camp Floyd Rogers*
Floyd Rogers Foundation
P.O. Box 31536
Omaha, NE 68131
402-341-0866

Contact: Sherman Poska
Residential camp and western camp

Camp Hot Shots*#
American Diabetes Association
Great Plains Region
7101 Newport Avenue, #207

Omaha, NE 68152
1-800-980-4932 or 402-496-5107

Contact: Cory Harter
Day camp

New Jersey
Camp Nejeda*#
Camp Nejeda Foundation
P.O. Box 156
Stillwater, NJ 07875-0156
973-383-2611

Contact: Valerie Miller
Residential camp/teen adventure
program/family session

New Mexico
Camp Challenge*#
American Diabetes Association
525 San Pedro, No. 101
Albuquerque, NM 87108
505-266-5716

Contact: Suzanne Miller
Residential camp

New York
Camp Carefree*
17 Washington Square
Albany, NY 12205
518-218-1755
603-659-7061

Contact: Beth Rowe

Camp Hagoo*
American Diabetes Association
Children's Hospital of Buffalo
Buffalo, NY 14222
716-878-7262
Residential camp

Camp Independence*#
Jewish Community Center of Staten Island
475 Victory Boulevard
Staten Island, NY 10301
718-317-1986

Contact: Susan Bernstein
Day camp

Camp LADD*#
Smith School
Wheeler Avenue

Cortland, NY
607-758-9086

Day camp

Camp Rainbow*#
American Diabetes Association
20 Ramona Street
Rochester, NY 14613
716-458-3040

Contact: Beverly Gaines
Residential/day camp

Camp Sunshine*#
American Diabetes Association
20 Ramona Street
Rochester, NY 14613
716-458-3040, Ext. 3475

Contact: Peggy Greenwalt/Charlene Mason
Residential camp

Circle of Life Camp, Inc.*
5 Woodridge Drive
Loudonville, NY 12211
518-459-3622

Residential camp

Holy Family Summer Camp*
25 Fordham Avenue
Hicksville, NY 11801
516-937-0636

Contact: Gary Turnier
Day camp

Lions Camp Badger*
Badger Diabetes Youth Camp
725 La Rue Road
Spencer, NY 14883
607-732-7069

Contact: Nancy
Residential camp

North Carolina
Camp Carolina Trails*#
American Diabetes Association
1820 East 7th Street
Charlotte, NC 28204
704-373-9111

Contact: Rick Bridges
Residential camp

Camp Coqui*
Graham Children's Medical Center
Mission St. Joseph's
509 Biltmore Avenue
Asheville, NC 28801

828-245-4701 or 1-800-377-9251

Residential camp

Camp Enscore*#
Diabetes Comprehensive Care Program
WFU Baptist Medical Center
Winston-Salem, NC 27157
704-373-9111, Ext. 3261

Contact: Diane Roth
Day camp

Camp Needles in Pines*
Department of Pediatrics
Brody Medical Sciences Building 3E-133
East Carolina University
School of Medicine
Greenville, NC 27858-4354
252-816-2516

Contact: Pam Hardy
Residential camp, ages 8–14

Cumberland County Day Camp*#
McPherson Presbyterian Church
3525 Clifdale Road
Fayetteville, NC 28304
910-485-5569

Contact: Sid Mozena/Heidi Mohn
Day camp, ages 5–14

Southern Region*
434 Fayetteville Street Mall
2 Hannover Square, Suite 1600
Raleigh, NC 27601
919-743-5400, Ext. 3201

North Dakota
Camp Sioux*
American Diabetes Association*
315 North Fourth Street
Grand Forks, ND 58206-5234
1-800-666-6709

Contact: Lynette Dickson
Residential camp, ages 8–14

Ohio
Camp CODA*
Central Ohio Diabetes Association
1580 King Avenue
Columbus, OH 43212-2058
614-486-7124

Day camp, ages 3–7

Camp Granada*#
217-875-9011

Contact: Donna Scott
Residential camp

Camp Hamwi*
Central Ohio Diabetes Association
1580 King Avenue
Columbus, OH 43212-2058
614-486-7124 or 1-800-422-7949

Contact: Darlene Honigford
Residential camp, ages 7–11; 11– 13; 14–17

Camp Ho Mita Koda*
Diabetes Association of Greater Cleveland
104 Auburn Road, Suite 100
Newbury, OH 44065
216-591-0800

Residential camp, ages 6–9; 9–12; 10–13;
13–15; Family mini-camp, ages 4–7
and parents

Camp Ko-man-she*
Diabetes Association of the Dayton Area
184 Salem Avenue
Dayton, OH 45406
947-220-6611

Contact: Bob Buckwalker
Residential camp, ages 6–12; 13–17

Camp Korelitz*#
American Diabetes Association
8899 Brookside Avenue, No. 102
West Chester, OH 45069
513-759-9330

Contact: Jill Honerlaw
Residential camp, ages 8–14

Camp Libbey*
Diabetes Youth Program
2238 Jefferson Avenue
Toledo, OH 43624
419-251-1796

Residential/day camp
Ages 10–15 (residential); 6–9 (day camp)

Camp Tokumto*#
American Diabetes Association
8899 Brookside Avenue, No. 102
West Chester, OH 45069
513-759-9330
Day camp, ages 5–9

Oklahoma
Camp Classen YMCA*
P.O. Box 1374
Oklahoma City, OK 73101
405-297-7740

Contact: Albert McWhorter
Residential camp, ages 8–15
Wranglers in training and Counselors in
Training, ages 16–17

Camp Endres*
American Diabetes Association
1211 North Sahrtel Avenue
Oklahoma City, OK 73104
405-949-6000

Contact: Kim Boaz
Residential camp, ages 9–16

Oregon
Chris Dudley Camp for Youth with Diabetes*
The Dudley Foundation
515 NW Saltzman Road, Suite 789
Portland, OR 97229
503-626-4007

Contact: Debbie Wakeman
Residential basketball camp

Gales Creek Camp*
American Diabetes Association
415 North State Street, No. 136
Lake Oswego, OR 97034-3231
503-699-8433

Contact: Patti Sadowski
Residential camp/family session

Pennsylvania
Camp Crestfield*#
1-800-676-4065

Contact: Terri Seidman
Residential camp

Camp Setebaid*#
Setebaid Services, Inc.
P.O. Box 196
Winfield, PA 17889
570-524-9090

Contact: Mark Moyer
Residential camp

Dr. Barclay Camp for
Diabetic Children at Camp Fitch
Hamot Diabetes Education Center*
300 State Street, Suite 304
Erie, PA 16550-0001

814-877-4690

Contact: Diane Harbough
Residential camp

Harrisburg Diabetic Youth Camp*#
11 Sycamore Lane
Palmyra, PA 17078-2839
570-524-9090

Contact: Mark Moyer
Residential camp

Kweebec & Wa-Shawtee Camps*
Camp Kweebec, Inc.
814 Woodbine Avenue, Box 511
Penn Valley, PA 19072
800-543-9830

Contact: Brett Rosenbloom
Residential camp

Southeast Pennsylvania*
1 Plymouth Meeting Street, Suite 520
Plymouth, PA 19462
610-828-5003, Ext. 4639

Southeast Pennsylvania*
1060 North Kings Street, #309
Cherry Hill, NJ 08034
856-482-9047, Ext. 3598

Puerto Rico
Cristo Redentor Camp*
Aguas, Puerto Rico
787-856-7950

Contact: Miriam Alicea
Residential camp

South Carolina
Camp Adam Fisher*#
American Diabetes Association
2711 Middleburg Drive
Kittrell Center, Suite 205
Columbia, SC 29204
800-342-2383

Contact: Debra Schmidt
Residential camp

Camp Independence*#
American Diabetes Association
P.O. Box 10794
Greenville, SC 29603

864-609-5054

Contact: Bridgette Adley
Day camp

South Dakota
Camp Gilbert*#
RR 1, Box 85
Wanbay, SD 57273
605-947-4440
Residential camp

Tennessee
Camp Easter Seals*
6300 Benders Ferry Road
Mount Juliet, TN 37122
615-444-2829

Contact: Jennifer Hargroves
Residential camp

Camp Hopewell*
154 East Harpers Herry Road
Collierville, TN 39017
901-853-1819 or 901-572-5036

Contact: Bob Trouy
Residential camp

Camp Rising Sun*
American Diabetes Association
6906 Kingston Pike, No. 201
Knoxville, TN 37919
423-584-0212

Contact: Rick Willis
Day camp

Camp Sugarbugs*
2354 Highway 41, Suite J
Greenbriar, TN 37073
615-643-9944
Residential camp

Camp Sugar Control*
Madison-Jackson County General Hospital
708 West Florida Avenue
Jackson, TN 38301
901-425-6665

Contact: Kathy Woolfork
Day camp

Camp Sugar Falls*#
American Diabetes Association
4205 Hillsboro Road, Suite 200
Nashville, TN 37215
615-298-3066

Contact: Melissa Schmittou
Day camp, ages 6–12

Tennessee Camp for Diabetic Children*
P.O. Box 4350
Chattanooga, TN 37405
432-843-5006

Contact: Rich Hidelgo
Residential camp

Texas
Camp Aurora*#
Fort Worth, TX
972-255-6900, Ext. 6012

Contact: Erika Flood
Day camp

Camp Bluebonnet*#
Specialty Care Center
Children's Hospital of Austin
601 East 15th Street
Austin, TX 78701
512-324-8864

Contact: Elizabeth Williams
Day camp

Camp New Horizons North*# and
Camp New Horizons South*#
4425 W. Airport Freeway, Suite 130
Irving, TX 75062
888-342-2383 Ext. 6097

Contact: Sherry Hill
Day camp

Camp Rainbow*#
American Diabetes Association
713-977-7706 Ext. 6085

Contact: Barbara Heame

Camp Sandcastle*#
Driscoll Children's Hospital
Diabetes Center
3533 South Alameda Street
Corpus Christi, TX 78411

Day camp

Camp Sweeny*
Southwestern Diabetic Foundation
P.O. Box 918
Gainesville, TX 76241
940-665-2011

Contact: Jay Murphy
Residential camp/mini session/
fall family session

Texas Lions Camp*
P.O. Box 247
Kerrville, TX 78029
830-896-8500

Contact: Steve Ponder/Susi Johnson
Residential camp

Utah
Camp UTADA*
American Diabetes Association
250 East 300 South, Suite 110
Salt Lake City, UT 84111
801-363-3024

Contact: Rob Birdsley
Residential camp

Vermont
Camp Carefree*#
207-685-4152

Contact: Helen Farrar
Residential camp

Virginia
Camp Holiday Trails*
P.O. Box 5806
Charlottesville, VA 22905-0806
804-977-3781

Contact: Bert Lippman
Residential camp

Camp Too Sweet*
700 Randolph Street
Radford, VA 24141
540-731-2645

Day camp

Chesapeake Health Diabetes Camps*
800 North Battlefield Street
Chesapeake, VA 23320
757-312-6132

Contact: Nancy Clark
Residential camp/day camp/
spring family session

Southern Region*
2015 Ivy Road, Suite 6
Charlottesville, VA 22903
804-974-9905

Washington
Black Lake Camp*
6521 Fairview Southwest
Olympia, WA 99114
206-282-4616, Ext. 7202

Contact: Laura Thelander
Residential camp

Camp Dudley*#
Yakima Family YMCA
P.O. Box 2885
Yakima, WA 98907
509-248-1202

Contact: Dustin Yaeger
Residential camp

Camp Leo Lions Camp*
28211 28th Avenue South
Federal Way, WA 98003
253-839-5418

Contact: Carol Malcom
Residential camp

Camp Orkila*#
YMCA
909 4th Avenue
Seattle, WA 98104
206-381-5009

Contact: Barbara Syre
Residential camp

Camp Sealth*#
8511 15th Avenue NE
Seattle, WA 98115
206-461-8550

Contact: Barbara Syre
Residential camp/fall family session

West Virginia
Camp Kno-Koma
Diabetes Camp of West Virginia
P.O. Box 1401
Charleston, WV 25325
304-346-1754

Contact: Jay Bowers
Residential camp

Wisconsin
Camp Lakoda*#
American Diabetes Association
2949 North Mayfair Road
Wauwatosa, WI 53222
414-778-5500, Ext. 190 or
888-342-2383

Residential camp

YMCA Camp St. Croix*
532 Country Road E
Hudson, WI 54016
651-436-8428

Contact: Jeanne Cloutier
Residential camp

Wyoming
Camp Colorado*
American Diabetes Association
Colorado/Wyoming/Montana Area
2480 West 26th Avenue, Suite 120B
Denver, CO 80210
720-855-1102, Ext. 7019

Residential camp/bike camp/
wilderness camp/equestrian camp

For camp listings in other countries, go to
www.diabetescamps.org/1n11camps.html
and www.diabetes.org/camp/diabetes camps
2003.pdf

Appendix K

Glossary of Diabetes-Related Terms

Acetoacetic acid An acid that also contains a ketone group in its molecule.

Acetone A ketone formed in greater abundance in the liver from fatty acids when glucose is not available to the cells for energy. Acetone, one of three ketones, is found in the blood and urine of people with uncontrolled diabetes and causes the breath to have a fruity odor.

Acidosis An acid condition of the body resulting from abnormal amounts of acid, such as acetoacetic and beta hydroxybutyric acids. Acidosis occurs in people who are not producing insulin or who do not receive enough insulin.

Adrenal glands Two tent-shaped organs that secrete epinephrine (see *epinephrine*) and glucocorticoids (see *glucocorticoids*) and aldosterone.

Adult diabetes Now called Type 2 or non-insulin-dependent diabetes mellitus. (See *Type 2 diabetes*.)

Alpha cells Cells that produce glucagon; found in the islets of Langerhans of the pancreas.

American Association of Diabetes Educators (AADE) A national voluntary organization of professionals interested in education of the person and/or family with diabetes.

American Diabetes Association, Incorporated (ADA) A national voluntary health organization of professional and lay people interested in research, service, and education in the field of diabetes.

American Dietetic Association (ADA).

Angiotensin converting enzyme (ACE) inhibitor. A medication known to improve the functioning of the kidneys (e.g., Acupril, Monopril).

Angiopathy Blood-vessel disease (see *microangiopathy* and *macroangiopathy*).

Antidiabetic agent A medication or herb that directly or indirectly affects blood-glucose levels.

Arteriosclerosis Thickening and hardening of the arteries due to fat buildup inside the blood vessels.

Aspartame An artificial sweetener, not usable for cooking.

Atrophy The shrinking of a body part due to lack of nutrition. In diabetes, this may mean a decrease in the amount of fat under the skin. This sometimes occurs at the sites of insulin injection and results in hollowed-out areas that are cosmetically undesirable.

Autonomic neuropathy Disease of the nerves that are not under conscious control of a person (e.g., erectile dysfunction).

Basement membrane Layers of concentric circles, or chains, of glycoproteins separated by infrequent glucose and galactose molecules, protectively surrounding cells of the capillaries of the kidneys, muscles, retina of the eye, etc.

BC-ADM Board Certified in Advanced Diabetes Management by the American Nurses Credentialing Center.

Beta cells Cells that produce insulin; found in the islet of Langerhans of the pancreas.

Beta hydroxybutyric acid One product of metabolized fat.

Biguanides Drugs, such as phenformin (DBI and DBI-TD), that have been used in the past in treating diabetes. They do not stimulate the pancreas to produce more insulin but prevent glucose uptake from the intestine, prevent gluconeogenesis (new glucose formation), and promote the breakdown of glucose, among other actions. Although these drugs are no longer available in the United States, a new phenformin called metformin is now available. It is found to be less of a cause of lactic acidosis, a side effect seen in the use of the earlier drugs, but is the major action of blocking glucose production in the liver.

Blood-glucose level The concentration of glucose in the blood. It is commonly called blood sugar and is usually measured in milligrams per deciliter (mg/dl) or in millimoles (mmol).

Blood-glucose meter A hand-held machine that tests blood-glucose levels. A drop of blood, obtained by pricking a finger, is placed on a small strip that is inserted in the meter, which calculates and displays the blood-glucose level.

Brittle diabetes A type of Type 1 diabetes in which the blood-glucose level fluctuates widely from high to low. Brittle diabetes can be caused by the complete loss of ability to produce any insulin, by too high an insulin dose, or by other factors. It can often be improved through a good treatment program. Also called *unstable diabetes.*

Callus A thickening of the skin caused by friction or pressure.

Calorie A unit for the measurement of heat. The heat-producing, or energy-producing, value of foods is measured in calories. A true calorie is such a small unit that 1,000 calories a kilocalorie is usually referred to as a calorie when discussing caloric values of food. In one dietary system, 75 calories is the equivalent of one point of food.

Calorie content The amount of heat released on the burning of 1 gram of food, most correctly called a kilocalorie (k).

Carbohydrate One of the three main constituents of foods. Carbohydrates are composed of sugars and starches. A measurement of 15 grams by a dietary program is equal to one carb point.

Cardiovascular disease Disease of the heart and large blood vessels; tends to occur more often and at a younger age in people with diabetes and may be related to how well the diabetes is controlled.

Cell membrane The material that surrounds all cells and acts to retain helpful substances, exclude harmful substances, and allow glucose to pass into the cells (with the help of insulin).

Certified Diabetes Educator (CDE) A health care professional who has passed an examination held by the National Board of Diabetes Education Certification.

Cesarean section An operation in which an infant is delivered by being removed from the mother's womb through an incision in the abdomen. Infants of diabetic mothers (IDMs) are frequently delivered before term by this means.

Charcot's joint Chronic progressive degeneration of the stress-bearing part of the foot (e.g., ankles, arches).

Cholesterol A mixture of lipoproteins found in blood, consisting of HDL (high-density lipoproteins), LDL (low-density lipoproteins), and VLDL (very-low-density lipoproteins). Present recommendations are to keep cholesterol levels below 200 mg/dl (11.1 mmol).

Closed-loop system A self-controlled blood-glucose control system (artificial pancreas or artificial beta cell).

Conventional control One, two, or three doses of insulin used to keep blood sugars in an acceptable but not in an ideal range, i.e., diabetes management sufficient enough to keep a person out of diabetic ketoacidosis.

Corns Hard, thickened areas of the skin caused by friction or pressure. These usually occur on the feet and may result in foot ulcers in people who have a loss of pain sensation in their feet.

Counter-regulatory hormones Hormones that directly or indirectly alter blood-glucose levels. All raise blood sugars except insulin, the only hormone that lowers blood-glucose levels. Often called stress hormones.

Creatinine A chemical in the blood and urine that indicates that the kidneys are functioning.

Dawn phenomenon An early morning rise in blood-glucose levels, believed to be due to a delayed response in growth-hormone release.

Diabetes Control and Complications Trial (DCCT) A ten-year research study sponsored by the National Institutes of Health (NIH) involving more than 1,400 people with Type 1 diabetes.

The study proved that tight blood-glucose control can prevent or delay diabetic complications related to hyperglycemia.

Diabetes mellitus A disease in which the body is unable to use and store glucose normally because of a decrease or lack of insulin production. Diabetes mellitus is usually inherited, but it may be caused by any process that destroys the pancreas (usually the beta cells) or alters the effectiveness of the receptor site on the cell membrane.

Diabetic coma Unconsciousness occurring during ketoacidosis. Associated symptoms include dry skin and mouth, fruity odor of the breath, very deep and rapid respirations, rapid pulse, and low blood pressure. Diabetic coma is caused by a deficiency of insulin.

Diabetic ketoacidosis (DKA) The most severe state of diabetes, in which there are markedly elevated glucose levels in blood and urine, elevated ketones in blood and urine, dehydration, and electrolyte imbalance. (See *ketoacidosis.*)

Diabetic ketosis A serious state of diabetes in which there is glucose in blood and urine, ketones in blood and urine, and possibly some dehydration. (See *ketosis.*)

Dialysis A method of washing the toxins out of the blood. Peritoneal dialysis is done at home (usually four hours in, four hours out); hemodialysis is done at home (usually twelve hours in, twelve hours out) or at a center.

Epinephrine A hormone released from the adrenal glands. Its main function in diabetes is to release glucose from the liver, increase the circulation rate, and prevent release of secreted insulin.

Exchange A serving of food that contains known and relatively constant amounts of carbohydrate, fat, and/or protein. The food used in an exchange is usually weighed or measured. The exchanges are divided into several groups: milk, fruit, meat, fat, bread, and vegetables.

Fasting blood glucose Blood-glucose concentration in the morning before breakfast. Commonly called fasting blood sugar (FBS).

Fat One of the three main constituents of foods. Fats occur in nearly pure form as liquids or solids, such as oils and margarines, or they may be a component of other foods. Fats may be of animal or vegetable origin. They have a higher energy content than any other food (9 calories per gram).

Fatty acids Constituents of fat. When there is an insulin deficiency, as in diabetes, fatty acids increase in the blood and are used by the liver to produce ketones.

Fiber Aids in the normal functioning of the digestive system, specifically the intestinal tract.

Flocculation A "snowy" look to insulin that may occur when the insulin has been exposed to too high or too low a temperature or when it is out of date.

Fluorescein angiopathy Procedure in which photographs of the retina are taken after a water-soluble dye has been injected into the vein.

Fractional urine Urine collected over a period of time and used to test for glucose and acetone levels. Fractions of urine are usually collected over twenty-four hours: from breakfast to lunchtime, from lunchtime to suppertime, from suppertime to bedtime, and from bedtime to rising. Also called block urine.

Fructose The sugar found mostly in fruits and some vegetables, used as a sweetener.

Gangrene The death of tissue caused by a very poor blood supply, as sometimes occurs in the feet and legs of persons with diabetes. Infection may be a contributing cause.

Genes Basic units of hereditary characteristics passed on through reproduction (part of chromosomes).

Gestational diabetes A period of abnormal glucose tolerance that occurs during pregnancy, usually controlled by diet and possibly insulin.

Globin insulin An early, developed, modified form of insulin produced by attaching a globin molecule to Regular insulin, slowing absorption and extending the peak and duration of action. Globin insulin was a clear insulin with acidic pH and intermediate action. It is no longer on the market.

Glucagon A hormone produced by the alpha cells in the islet of Langerhans of the pancreas. Glucagon causes a rise in the blood-glucose level by releasing stored glucose from liver and muscle cells. It is given by injection for the treatment of severe insulin reactions at home, school, or work (1 mg for those over age five; ½ mg for children ages three to five; ¼ mg for children under three years of age). The major side effect is nausea that usually lasts for only a short period of time.

Glucocorticoids Hormones released from the cortex of the adrenal gland; in relation to diabetes, they cause amino acids to be changed into new glucose (gluconeogenesis).

Gluconeogenesis The process of converting amino acids and glycerol into new glucose. This process takes place in the liver and muscle cells of the body.

Glucose The simple sugar, also known as dextrose, that is found in the blood and is used by the body for energy.

Glucose sensor An instrument worn for three days to determine blood-glucose patterns around the clock.

Glucose tolerance The ability of the body to use and store glucose. Glucose tolerance is zero in persons with diabetes mellitus.

Glucose-tolerance test A test for diabetes mellitus. The person being tested is given a measured amount of glucose to drink; blood-glucose levels are measured before ingestion and one-half, one-and-a-half, two, three, and sometimes four to six hours after ingestion. Also called oral glucose tolerance test (OGTT).

Glucose toxicity A state in which the lack of insulin, due to a decreased availability and/or function of the cell receptor site to receive insulin, results in an increase of glucose in the body, which is toxic to the beta cells in the islet of Langerhans. This toxicity is such that it may even lead to beta cell death.

Gluco-Watch A device sensitive to blood-glucose levels, with an alarm for too-low and too-high blood sugars.

Glycogen Glucose in storage form in the liver. It may be broken down to form blood glucose during an insulin reaction or during a fast.

Glycogenesis The process whereby the liver converts a portion of glucose to glycogen.

Glycogenolysis The breakdown of glycogen to glucose.

Glycohemoglobin A test that reflects average blood-glucose control for about two to three months prior to the time of the test. One of these tests is the commonly used hemoglobin A1c.

Glycolysis The breakdown of glucose into carbon dioxide and water.

Glycosuria The presence of glucose in the urine (*glyco* refers to sugar, *uria* to urine).

Gram A small unit of weight in the metric system. Used in weighing food to determine a specific amount to eat or to burn in calories (1 pound, or 16 ounces, equals 453 grams).

Health care team The group of professionals who help manage diabetes and which may include a physician, registered dietitian, certified diabetes educator, ophthalmologist, podiatrist, or other specialists.

Heart disease A cardiovascular condition in which the heart does not efficiently pump blood. People with diabetes are at greater risk for developing heart disease than is the general population.

Hemoglobin A1c Measures the percent of glucose attached to the protein in the red blood cells (life span of a red blood cell is about 120 days or two to three months). Knowing this number in the nondiabetic population aids in managing abnormal blood glucose to attain the same percentages.

Heredity The transmission of a trait, such as blue eyes, from parents to offspring.

Hormone A chemical substance produced by one gland or tissue and carried by the blood to other tissues or organs, where it stimulates action and causes a specific effect. Insulin and glucagon are hormones.

Human insulin A synthetic insulin that is similar to insulin produced by the body.

Hyperbilirubinemia Condition in which a person has greater-than-normal value (+12.50 mg/dl in the infant) of bilirubin in the blood. Signs are jaundiced look to skin and whites of eyes.

Hyperglycemia A greater-than-normal level of glucose in the blood (high blood glucose). Fasting blood-glucose values greater than 105 mg/dl (5.8 mmol) are suspect; greater than 140 mg/dl (7.8 mmol) are diagnostic.

Hyperinsulinism An excessive amount of insulin, which may be caused by overproduction of insulin by the beta cells of the islets of Langerhans in the pancreas or by an excessive dose of insulin. Hyperinsulinism may cause hypoglycemia (low blood-glucose levels).

Hyperlipidemia Elevated fats or lipids in the blood (LDL, low-density lipoprotein, should be less than 100; HDL, high-density lipoprotein, should be greater than 45).

Hypertension High blood pressure. Found to aggravate diabetes control or the complications already developed.

Hypocalcemia Less-than-normal value (10 to 12 mg/dl in the infant) of calcium in the blood. Signs are convulsive seizure and irritability of the neuromuscular system.

Hypoglycemia A less-than-normal level of glucose in the blood (low blood-glucose level). Fasting blood-glucose value less than 60 mg/dl (3.3 mmol).

Hypoglycemic agent A drug or substance, such as sulfonylureas (e.g., Tolbutamide) and glipizide, used to reduce blood-glucose levels.

IDF International Diabetes Federation.

Impaired glucose tolerance Condition that exists when blood-glucose values are elevated above normal but are inconclusive for diabetes. Sometimes mistakenly called borderline diabetes.

Implantable insulin pump Pump placed inside the body for the delivery of insulin and controlled internally by a battery and externally by a transmitter.

Insulin A hormone secreted by the beta cells of the islets of Langerhans in the pancreas. Promotes the utilization of glucose.

Insulin binding An external device that delivers a small amount of insulin every few minutes.

Insulin-dependent diabetes mellitus An older term, along with juvenile diabetes, now called Type 1 diabetes.

Insulin pump An external device that delivers a small amount of insulin every few minutes (basal rate) and manually or automatically delivers boluses of insulin depending on food eaten or to be eaten.

Insulin reaction A condition with rapidly occurring onset that is the result of low blood-glucose levels. It may be caused by too much insulin, too little food, or an increase in exercise without a corresponding increase in food or decrease in insulin. Symptoms may vary from nervousness, shakiness, headaches, and drowsiness to confusion and convulsions, and even to coma.

Insulin resistance A condition in which the body does not properly respond to insulin. It is the most common cause of Type 2 diabetes.

Intensive control Three or more doses of insulin per day or use of an insulin infusion pump, with blood sugars in the normal or near-normal range 80 percent or more of the time.

International Society for Pediatric and Adolescent Diabetes (ISPAD)

Islets of Langerhans The small groups of cells in the pancreas that contain alpha, beta, and delta cells and reduce glucagon, insulin, and somatostatin.

Isophane insulin NPH (neutral protamine Hagedorn) insulin, a neutral pH, intermediate-acting insulin.

Juvenile diabetes Now called Type 1 rather than insulin-dependent diabetes mellitus.

Juvenile Diabetes Foundation (JDF).

Ketoacidosis A condition of the body in which there is not enough insulin. Free fatty acids are released from fat cells and produce ketones in the liver. These ketones or acids result in an imbalance of the blood (acidosis). In the more acute state, the result is ketoacidosis. Large amounts of sugar and ketones are found in urine, electrolytes are imbalanced, and dehydration is present. The onset is usually slow. The condition leads to loss of appetite, abdominal pain, nausea and vomiting, rapid and deep respiration, and coma. Death may occur.

Ketone bodies A name given by some to a mixture of ketones and other metabolism products that may break down into ketones. These other metabolism products are usually acetoacetic acid (which has a ketone group within the molecule) and beta hydroxybutyric acid (a molecule very similar to acetoacetic acid).

Ketonemia The presence of ketones in the blood.

Ketones Substances formed in the blood when a fat is broken down because of insufficient insulin. Fats are broken down into fatty acids, which are then chemically changed into ketones. Ketones (usually acetone) are often found in the blood and urine of persons with uncontrolled diabetes. Ketones may produce a fruity odor in the breath and urine of a person.

Ketonuria The presence of ketones in the urine.

Ketosis The presence of large amounts of ketones in the body, secondary to excessive breakdown of fat caused by insufficient insulin in a person with diabetes mellitus. Acidosis precedes and causes ketosis; the combination (ketosis and acidosis) is called ketoacidosis. Ketosis can also result from starvation or illness in nondiabetic individuals.

Kidney (or renal) threshold The level of a substance (such as glucose) in the blood in the kidney, above which it will be spilled into the urine.

Kimmelstiel-Wilson syndrome Lesions of the filtered tubules of the kidney, caused by blood-vessel degeneration related to poorly controlled diabetes, as described by doctors Kimmelstiel and Wilson.

Kussmaul's respiration The rapid, deep, and labored respiration observed in patients with diabetic ketoacidosis; an involuntary mechanism to excrete carbon dioxide in order to reduce carbonic-acid level.

Labile diabetes A term used for unstable diabetes control. (See *brittle diabetes*.)

Lente insulin An intermediate-acting insulin that is a mixture of 30 percent Semilente (not available since 1994) and 70 percent Ultralente insulin.

Lipolysis The increased fat breakdown in the body tissues that occurs in ketosis (lysis of fat).

Liver activation treatment Pulsatile intravenous insulin treatment. Insulin given by vein in a pulselike fashion (insulin based on total body needs given in short spurts every few seconds while the person sips a high glucose–loaded drink).

Macroangiopathy Disease related to the large blood vessels of the body.

Maturity-onset diabetes The older name for Type 2 diabetes (also called adult diabetes, non-insulin-dependent diabetes, mild diabetes, and ketone-resistant diabetes).

Mauriac syndrome A condition observed before puberty in children with prolonged, poorly controlled diabetes. It involves an enlarged, fatty liver, pitting edema, and short stature. The Mauriac syndrome is seldom seen today due to proper treatment, with adequate food and insulin provided for growth.

Meal plan An arrangement whereby the total food allowed daily is expressed in terms of a certain number of points or exchanges, with the foods to be eaten at specific times.

Metabolism All the chemical processes in the body, including those by which foods are broken down and used for tissue or energy production.

mg/dl Milligrams per deciliter. The unit of measure used to describe blood-glucose levels.

Microaneurysms Small ballooned-out areas on the capillary blood vessels, such as might be found on the retina of the eye. They may burst and bleed.

Microangiopathy Disease related to the small blood vessels of the body.

Monounsaturated fat Has effect similar to that of polyunsaturated fat but does not lower HDL cholesterol. Found in olive oil and other oils.

NDEP National Diabetes Education Program. Promotes efforts to improve the caliber of education for both professionals and the public.

Nephropathy Disease of the kidneys that can be life threatening.

Neuritis Inflammation of the nerves.

Neutral protamine Hagedorn (NPH) An intermediate-acting insulin that initially received its slower action through the addition of a protein to short-acting insulin.

Neuropathy Any disease of the nervous system. Neuropathy may occur in persons with diabetes. Polyneuropathy (many nerve diseases) is related to poor control of blood sugars. Mononeuropathy (one nerve disease, e.g., Bell's palsy) is not found to be related to blood-glucose levels, but occurs more frequently in people with diabetes. Symptoms such as pain, loss of sensation, loss of reflexes, and/or weakness may occur.

Non-insulin-dependent diabetes The old name for Type 2 diabetes.

Non-invasive blood-glucose monitoring Focuses on measuring blood sugars without having to damage the skin.

Obesity An abnormal and excessive amount of body fat. Obesity is a risk factor for Type 2 diabetes.

Omega Three fatty acids that are useful in lowering triglycerides and cholesterol. They also slow blood clotting. Found in salmon, tuna, and certain other fish.

Open-loop system A mechanical system of insulin injection that is not self-controlled but must be controlled or programmed externally.

Oral agents (oral hypoglycemic agents) Medications in pill form taken orally to lower blood glucose. They are used by people with Type 2 diabetes and should not be confused with insulin. (See *hypoglycemic agent.*)

Oral glucose-tolerance test (OGGT) (See *glucose-tolerance test.*)

Pancreas A gland that is positioned near the stomach and that secretes at least two hormones insulin and glucagon and many digestive enzymes.

Pancreas, artificial A mechanical device that stimulates the functions of the beta cells. It withdraws blood continuously, measures the glucose level, and injects an appropriate dose of insulin or glucose to reestablish a normal blood-glucose level.

Pancreas transplant Replacing part or all of a pancreas with a donor pancreas from a family member or cadaver.

Podiatrist A health professional who has completed four years of education focusing solely on foot diseases and other problems related to the feet.

Points system A method of quantifying food intake by assigning points to various food components (carbohydrate, fat, protein, calories, sodium, etc.) and determining the number of each component point needed for a meal or for a day's intake. This system may either substitute for or accompany the less precise exchange system for diet calculations (75 calories = 1 point).

Polydipsia Excessive thirst, with increased drinking of water.

Polyphagia Excessive hunger or appetite, resulting in increased food intake.

Polyunsaturated fat The type of fat that is liquid at room temperature, unless hydrogenated. Includes corn and certain other vegetable oils.

Polyuria Excessive output of urine.

Postprandial Occurring after a meal.

Potential abnormality of glucose tolerance The time during the life of a diabetic person before any abnormality in glucose tolerance can be demonstrated. The identical twin of a person with diabetes is thought to have potential abnormality of glucose tolerance.

Precipitate Particles that settle out of solution. This may occur in insulin that is kept beyond the expiration date, is contaminated, or is improperly mixed.

Prediabetes Previously called impaired glucose tolerance or impaired glucose homeostatis.

Previous abnormality of glucose tolerance A classification used for the person who has been documented to have hyperglycemia during pregnancy, illness, or other crisis but who currently has relatively normal blood-glucose levels without any treatment.

Protamine zinc insulin (PZI) A long-acting insulin, prepared with large amounts of protamine combined with Regular insulin in the presence of zinc.

Protein One of the three main constituents of foods. Proteins are made up of amino acids and are found in foods such as milk, meat, fish, and eggs. Proteins are essential constituents of all living cells and are the nitrogen-containing nutrient. The caloric content of protein is 4 calories per gram.

Regular insulin Short-acting insulin crystallized from the pancreas of animals or synthetically made. This insulin is neutralized and can be premixed with NPH insulin. Also known as clear insulin or crystalline insulin.

Renal Pertaining to the kidneys.

Renal threshold Another name for kidney threshold.

Respiratory distress syndrome (RDS) Difficulty in breathing, noted by grunting, respiratory or expiratory wheezing or both, labored respiration, cyanosis (a blueness of the lips, face, fingers, and toes that can expand to involve the total body), and abnormal rate of respiration.

Retina The light-sensitive layer at the back of the inner surface of the eyeball.

Retinopathy Disease of the retina. Retinopathy occurs in persons with prolonged, poorly controlled diabetes and involves abnormal growth of and bleeding from the capillary blood vessels in the eye.

Saturated fat The type of fat, such as butter, that is usually solid at room temperature. Saturated fats are usually derived from animal sources.

Self-monitoring of blood glucose (SMBG) A technique of testing a person's blood-glucose level in order to determine the body's response to activity, food, and medication.

Semilente Insulin prepared through special crystallizing techniques to produce small insulin crystals with large absorptive surfaces and rapid action. Semilente is slower in action than Regular insulin but more rapid than the intermediate-acting insulin. This insulin is no longer on the market.

Serum glucose The concentration of glucose in the liquid part of the blood after the cells have been removed (clotted blood).

Single-void technique The procedure of collecting a urine specimen.

Somogyi effect A phenomenon (described by the biochemist Somogyi) in which hypoglycemia causes activation of the internal counterregulatory hormones (for example, glucagon, growth hormone, and epinephrine), causing a rebound in the blood-glucose level to hyperglycemic levels. Also called posthypoglycemia hyperglycemia.

Spot test A urine test performed on a sample collected using the single-void technique.

Sugar A form of carbohydrate that provides calories and raises blood glucose levels.

Sugar substitutes Sweeteners, such as saccharin, acesulfame K, and aspartame, that are used as a substitute for sugar.

Sulfonylureas Chemical compounds that stimulate production or release of insulin by the beta cells in the pancreas and/or prevent release of glucose from the liver. They are used in the treatment of Type 2 diabetes.

Time-action curve A curve that shows the effect of a medicine at various times after it is administered.

Twenty-four-hour (or twelve-hour) urine Used to measure quantitative glucose or protein levels in urine from a pooled, twenty-four-hour specimen. Often used to calculate creatinine clearance or the ability to pass urine through the kidneys.

Type 1 diabetes Results from inability to make insulin due to a combination of genetics or inheritance and environmental stressors. Insulin-dependent diabetes mellitus is associated with insulin's lack of availability, its action on the receptor sites, and/or its function with the glycolytic pathway. Older names were insulin-dependent diabetes or juvenile diabetes.

Type 2 diabetes A type of diabetes that is usually found in adults over thirty years of age. The onset is gradual, and the symptoms are often minimal. Patients are often overweight. Those with Type 2 are less prone to acute complications, such as acidosis and coma, than are patients with Type 1. Type 2 diabetes is treated through diet alone or through diet plus oral hypoglycemic agents. Insulin injections may or may not be required. Older names were non-insulin-dependent diabetes, non-ketosis-prone diabetes, or maturity-onset diabetes. Previously called adult diabetes or maturity-onset diabetes in the young (MODY).

Ultralente A long-acting insulin that is prepared using special crystallizing techniques that produce large crystals with small absorptive surfaces. Similar but not as long acting as the old PZI.

Unsaturated fats The type of fat, such as vegetable oil, that is usually liquid at room temperature. (See *monounsaturated fat, polyunsaturated fat,* and *saturated fat.*)

Unstable diabetes Another name for brittle diabetes.

Urine tests Tests that measure substances in the urine. They provide a general idea of a patient's blood-glucose level several hours before the test. Urine tests for ketones are important for early recognition of the possibility of ketoacidosis.

Vitrectomy The removal and replacement of the gel found in the center of the eyeball.

Xylitol A substitute for sugar that contains some calories.

Appendix L

Diabetes-Related Websites

Diana Guthrie www.homeearthlink/~dianaguthrie

Abbott Laboratories;
  MediSense Products www.abbott.com

Activa Brand Products, Inc. www.advantajet.com

Alternative and
  Complementary
  Information (government) www.nccam.nih.gov

Alternative and
  Complementary
  Information www.alternativediabetes.com

American Association of
  Diabetes Educators www.aadenet.org

American Diabetes
  Association www.diabetes.org

Amira Medical www.amira.com

Animas Insulin Pump www.animascorp.com

Aventis Pharmaceuticals www.aventispharma_us.com

Bayer Corporation
  Diagnostics Division www.glucometer.com

BD (Becton Dickinson) www.bd.com/diabetes

Bioject, Inc. www.bioject.com

Bristol-Myers Squibb www.bmx.com

Canadian Diabetes
  Association www.diabetes.ca

Can-Am Care Corp. www.invernessmedical.com

Cell Robotics Inc. www.cellrobotics.com

Centers for Disease Control
   Diabetes Home Page   www.cdc.gov/nccdphp/ddt/
      ddthome.html
Children with Diabetes   www.childrenwithdiabetes.com
Diabetes   www.nd.edu/~hhowisen/
      diabetes.html
Diabetes Bookstore   www.merchant.diabetes.org
Diabetes Camping Association   www.diabetescamp.org
Diabetes.com   www.diabetes.com
Diabetes Forecast   www.diabetes.org/diabetesforecast
Diabetes Game for
   Children with Diabetes   www.starbright.org
Diabetes Guide to the
   Internet—Diabetes   www.pslgroup.com/diabetes.html
Diabetes in America, 2nd ed.   www.diabetes-in-
      america.s3.com/default.html
Diabetes in Control   www.diabetesincontrol.com
Diabetes Information at
   Mediconsult.com   www.mediconsult.com/diabetes
Diabetes Monitor, Page One   www.mdcc.com
Diabetes One Stop   www.diabetesonestop.com
Diabetes Self-Management
   magazine   www.diabetes-self-mgmt.com
Diabetes World   www.diabetesworld.com
Disetronic Medical
   Systems, Inc.   www.disetronic_usa.com
Eli Lilly & Company   www.lilly.com
Equidyne Systems, Inc.   www.equidyne.com
Home Diagnostics, Inc.   www.hdidiabetes.com
ICN Pharmaceuticals, Inc.   www.instaglucose.com
I.D. Technology, Inc.   www.id_technology.com
Identi-Find   www.identifind.com
Insuleeve   www.insuleeve.com
Joslin Diabetes Center   www.joslin.org
Juvenile Diabetes
   Foundation International   www.jdfcure.com
LifeScan, Inc.   www.lifescan.com
Lighthouse Catalog   www.lighthouse.org

Managing Your Diabetes	www.lilly.com/diabetes
Metrika, Inc.	www.a1cnow.com
Mid America Diabetes Associates	www.madiabetes.com
MedicAlert Foundation	www.medicalert.org
Medi-Ject Corporation	www.mediject.com
MiniMed, Inc.	www.minimed.com
National Institutes of Diabetes, Digestive and Kidney Diseases	www.niddk.nih.gov/ niddk_homepage.html
Novo-Nordisk Pharmaceuticals, Inc.	www.novo-nordisk.com
Online Diabetes	www.onlinediabetes.com
Pharmacia + Upjohn Company	www.pnu.com
Professional education internet course	www.twsu.edu/!wsucothp/n733
Professionals working with children	www.professionals@ childrenwithdiabetes.com
Roche Diagnostics	www.roche.com www.accu-chek.com
SmithKline Beecham Pharmaceuticals	www.sb.com
Takeda Pharmaceuticals America, Inc.	www.takedapharm.com
Wal-Mart Stores, Inc., Corporate Offices	www.childrenwithdiabetes. com/relion
Wizdom (for kids)	www.diabetes.org/wizdom

Bibliography

Chapter 1 What Kind of Diabetes Do You Have?

American Diabetes Association. "Report of the Expert Committee on the Diagnosis and Classification of Diabetes Mellitus." *Diabetes Care* 26, Suppl.1 (2001): S5–S20.

Clark, W. "What's Your Type?" *Diabetes Self-Management* (May/June 2001): 99–103.

The Diabetes Dictionary, rev. ed. Washington, D.C.: U.S. Dept. of Health and Human Services (National Diabetes Information Clearinghouse). NIH Pub. No. 89-3016, 1998.

Diabetes Facts and Figures, 2003. Accessed at www.diabetes.org/ada/facts.asp.

Fischman, J. "The Diabetes Epidemic: A Killer Disease—And How Diet and Lifestyle Can Help Beat It." *US News*, 25 June 2001, 59–61, 64–68.

"Number Crunching Diabetes." *Diabetes Self-Management* (November/December, 1999): 16–17.

Chapter 2 Who Gets This Disease?

101 Tips for Staying Healthy with Diabetes. Alexandria, Va.: American Diabetes Association, 1996.

American Diabetes Association. *Diabetes Statistics 2001*.

"Diabetes Update." RN 64 (2001): 59–64.

"Famous Diabetics." *Diabetes Interview* (June 1999): 34.

Saudek, C. D., and S. Margolis. *The Johns Hopkins White Papers: Diabetes Mellitus*. Baltimore, Md.: The Johns Hopkins Medical Institutions, 2003.

Chapter 3 How Is Diabetes Treated?

American Diabetes Association. "Standards of Medical Care for Patients with Diabetes Mellitus." *Diabetes Care* 26, Suppl. 1 S33–S50 (2003): 5.

Guber, C. *Type 2 Diabetes Life Plan: Take Charge, Take Care and Feel Better Than Ever.* New York: Broadway Books, 2002.

Guthrie, D. W., and R. A. Guthrie. *Nursing Management of Diabetes Mellitus: A Guide to the Pattern Approach.* 5th ed. New York: Spring Publishing Co., 2002.

Chapter 4 What About Education?

American Diabetes Association. "Third-Party Reimbursement of Diabetes Care, Self-Management Education, and Supplies." *Diabetes Care* 26, Suppl. 1 (2001): S143–S144.

Diabetes A to Z: *What You Need to Know About Diabetes Simply Put.* 4th. ed. Alexandria, Va.: American Diabetes Association, 1996.

An Educational Curriculum for Diabetes Camps. Franklin Lakes, N.J.: Becton Dickinson Consumer Products, 1997.

"Resource Guide 2003: Buyer's Guide." *Diabetes Forecast* (January 2003).

Chapter 5 How Should You Eat?

American Diabetes Association: *Month of Meals: Meals in Minutes,* 3rd ed. Alexandria, Va.: American Diabetes Association, 2003.

American Diabetes Association/American Dietetic Association. Diabetic Exchanges: *The Official Pocket Guide.* Alexandria, Va.: American Diabetes Association, 1999.

Brackenridge, B. P., and R. D. Rubin. *Sweet Kids: How to Balance Diabetes Control and Good Nutrition with Family Peace.* 2nd ed. Alexandria, Va.: American Diabetes Association, 2002.

Challem, J., B. Berkson, and M. D. Smith. *Syndrome X: The Complete Nutritional Program to Prevent and Reverse Insulin Resistance.* New York: John Wiley & Sons, Inc., 2000.

Friesen, J., N. Herring, and S. Reichenberger. *Points in Your Favor.* 7th ed. Wichita, Kans.: Via Christi–St. Joseph Campus, 2000.

Karpf, J., and J. Hazlet. "What Your Doctor Is Reading: Vitamins." *Diabetes Self-Management* 19, no. 5 (2002): 42–48.

Keane, M., and D. Chace. *What to Eat If You Have Diabetes: A Guide to Adding Nutritional Therapy to Your Treatment Plan.* Chicago: Contemporary Books, 1999.

Trecochi, D., and J. Roszler. "Herbs, Supplements and Vitamins: What to Try, What to Buy." *Diabetes Interviews* 11, no. 10 (2002): 49–56.

Warshaw, H. *Complete Guide to Carb Counting*. Alexandria, Va.: American Diabetes Association, 2002.

Chapter 6 What About Medications?

American Diabetes Association. "2003 Resource Guide." *Diabetes Forecast* (January 2003).

Bliss, M. *The Discovery of Insulin*. Chicago: University of Chicago Press, 1982.

Brackenridge, B. P., and R. O. Dolinar. Diabetes 101: *A Pure and Simple Guide for People Who Use Insulin*. 2nd ed. Minneapolis, Minn.: Chronimed Publishers, Inc., 1996.

Inzucchi, S. E. "Metformin or Thoazolidinediories as First-Line Therapy in Type 2 Diabetes." *Practical Diabetologs* 21, no. 3 (2002): 7–12.

Lindholm, A., et al. "Improved Glycemic Control with Insulin as Part: A Randomized Double-Blind Crossover Trial in Type 1 Diabetes Mellitus." *Diabetes Care* 22 (1999): 801–5.

Trecroci, D. "One-Shot-a-Day Insulin Is Here: Physicians Tout Lantus, Calling It Advancement in Basal Insulin Coverage." *Diabetes Interview* (2001): 41, 46.

Chapter 7 What Is Important About Exercise?

Graham, C., J. Biermann, and B. Toohey. *The Diabetic Sports and Exercise Book*. Los Angeles: Lowell House, 1996.

Richardson, D. "Exercise Your Right to a Healthy Body." *Diabetes Forecast* (August 2001): 65–67.

Trecroci, D. "Why People Quit: Exercise Physiologist Says Behavior Model May Explain Why People Don't Stick to Workout Regimens." *Diabetes Interview* (March 2001): 25–27.

Weil, R. "Obesity, Type 2 Diabetes, and Physical Activity (Includes Body Mass Index Chart)." *Diabetes Self-Management* (May/June 2001): 39–51.

Chapter 8 What About Hygiene?

Diabetes: Dental Tips. National Diabetes Information Clearing-house, DM–16, 2001.

Diabetes and Periodontal Disease: Guide for Patients. National Diabetes Information Clearinghouse, DM–21, 2001.

Saudeck, C.D., and S. Margolis. In *The Johns Hopkins White Papers on Diabetes* (2003): 33–34.

Tanenberg, R. M., and M. A. Pfeifer. "Fend Off Foot Ulcers." *Diabetes Forecast* (August 2001): 86–89.

Chapter 9 How Is Diabetes Monitored?

Getting Started: Urine Testing for Ketones. Franklin Lakes, N.J.: Becton Dickinson, 1995.

Patterned Diabetes Care. Eli Lilly & Co., 1998.

Goldstein, D. "For Parents: Setting Blood Glucose Goals." *Diabetes Self-Management* (May/June 2001): 94–97.

Nakamoto, M. "Software Options for *Diabetes Management* (Includes Charts on Blood Glucose Monitoring Software, Nutrient and Meal Planning Software, and Internet-Based Programs)." *Diabetes Self-Management* (May/June 2001): 61–72.

"Recent Progress in Glycohemoglobin (Hb A1c) Testing." *Diabetes Care* 23 (2000): 265–66.

Chapter 10 What Are the Possible Complications of Diabetes?

American Diabetes Association. *Keeping Your Heart Healthy Despite Diabetes.* Alexandria, Va.: American Diabetes Association, 2002.

Ahroni, J. *IDI Foot Care Tips for People with Diabetes.* Alexandria, Va.: American Diabetes Association, 2002.

Curtis, J. L. *Living with Diabetes Complications.* Shippensburg, Pa.: Companion Press, 1993.

D'Arrigo, T. "Ketoacidosis: The Snake in the Grass." *Diabetes Forecast* (July 2001): 70–74.

Levin, M. E., and M. A. Pfeiffer, eds. *The Uncomplicated Guide to Diabetic Complications.* Alexandria, Va.: American Diabetes Association, 1998.

Prevention Series. *Prevent Diabetes Problems.* National Diabetes Information Clearinghouse, DM 203-209, 2001.

Understanding Gestational Diabetes. National Diabetes Information Clearinghouse, DM–27, 2001.

Chapter 11 How Do You Adjust to Having Diabetes?

Creekmore, C. *Zen and the Art of Diabetes Maintenance.* Alexandria, Va.: American Diabetes Association, 2002.

International Diabetes Center. *Diabetes and Depression.* Minneapolis, Minn.: International Diabetes Center, 2002.

Polansky, W. H. *Diabetes Burnout: What to Do If You Can't Take It Anymore.* Alexandria, Va.: American Diabetes Association, 1999.

Rapaport, W. S. *When Diabetes Hits Home.* Alexandria, Va.: American Diabetes Association, 1997.

Rubin, R. R., J. Biermann, and B. Toohey. *Psyching Out Diabetes.* 2nd ed. Los Angeles: Lowell House, 1997.

Winning with Diabetes: A Diabetes Forecast Book. Alexandria, Va.: American Diabetes Association, 1997.

Chapter 12 How Does Stress Affect Diabetes?

Beating Stress (pamphlet). Alexandria, Va.: American Diabetes Association, 1996.

Caring for the Diabetic Soul. Alexandria, Va.: American Diabetes Association, 1997.

Feste, C. *Meditations on Diabetes: Strengthening Your Spirit in Every Season.* Alexandria, Va.: American Diabetes Association, 1999.

Rubin, R. R. "Diabetes and Stress." *Diabetes Wellness Letter* 6 (2000): 1–2, 8.

Siminerio, L. M. "When Your Preschooler Has Diabetes." *Diabetes Forecast* (September 1996): 59–60.

Youngs, B. B. *Stress and Your Child: Helping Kids Cope with the Strains and Pressures of Life.* New York: Fawcett/Columbine, 1995.

Chapter 13 How Can You Help Your Health Care Team Help You?
A Guide for You and Your Diabetes Care Team. Alexandria, Va.:
    American Diabetes Association, (order code 5983-06), 2001.
American Diabetes Association's Complete Guide to Diabetes,
    3rd ed. Alexandria, Va.: American Diabetes Association, 2002.
Testing Your Glucose Level (pamphlet). Alexandria, Va.: American
    Diabetes Association, 1996.

Chapter 14 How Can You Help Your Family and Friends Help You?
Barrett, J. "Diagnosis: Diabetes: For Parents and Families Learning
    to Cope the First Year." *JDRF Countdown* 22 (Summer
    2001): 34–39.
Biermann, J., and B. Toohey. *The Diabetic's Book: All Your Ques-
    tions Answered*. 4th ed. New York: G. P. Putnam's Sons, 1998.
Kruger, D. *The Diabetes Travel Guide*. Alexandria, Va.: American
    Diabetes Association, 2002.
NurrieStearns, R., and M. West. *Soulful Living: The Process of
    Personal Transformation*. Deerfield Beach, Fla.: Health
    Communications, Inc., 1999.

**Chapter 15 What Is Being Done to Conquer Diabetes and Improve
    Its Management?**
Chase, H. P., and M. D. Roberts. "Moms and Dads Take Note:
    Continuous Glucose Monitoring Is Coming." *Diabetes
    Interview* (June 2001): 46–49.
Culverwell, M. "Retinopathy Realities." *JDRF Countdown* 22,
    no. 3 (2001): 48–52.
Guthrie, D. *Alternative and Complementary Diabetes Care: How
    to Combine Natural and Traditional Therapies*. New York:
    John Wiley & Sons, Inc., 2000.
Juvenile Diabetes Research Foundation (JDRF). "Research in
    the Midst of a Milestone." *JDRF Countdown* 23, no. 4
    (2002): 40–46.
Spiegel, A. M. "Where We Stand with Research & Prevention
    at the National Institutes of Health." *Diabetes Interview*
    (April 2001): 23–27.
Trecroci, D. "GlucoWatch Approved." *Diabetes Interview*
    (May 2001): 2, 30–31, 34–35.

Index

acarbose (Precose), 57–58
acetohexamide (Dymelor), 55
Actos, 58, 59, 170. *See also*
    thiazolidinediones (TZDs)
acute care, Type 1 diabetes, 25–26
ADA Forecast, 105, 109
adrenaline release, 139, 140
advanced patterned management,
    102–3
aerobic exercise, 78–79
age
    diabetes and, 5
    exercise and, 84
    heart disease and, 129
    skin condition and, 87
aging
    control of diabetes and, 27, 30
    renal thresholds and, 98
Albolene, 92
algorithm approach to insulin
    management, 100, 101–2
alpha glucosidase inhibitors, 52, 54,
    57–58
alternative health care choices,
    158–59
Amaryl, 55, 57
American Association of Diabetes
    Educators, 36, 37, 97
American Association of Sex
    Educators, Counselors, and
    Therapists, 92
American Diabetes Association
    (ADA), 24, 31, 97, 158,
    172, 173
American Heart Association, 42
American Medical Association, 146
American Nurses Certification
    Corporation (ANCC), 37

amputation, 3
anaerobic exercise, 79–80
analogue insulins, 39
angiotensin converting enyzme
    (ACE), 127, 129
antidepressants, 124
antihyperglycemic agents, 57–59
arteriosclerosis, 130
artificial transplants, 162–64
aspart (Novolog), 28, 29, 64
    See also Novolog
attitude, toward diabetes, 142
autogenic therapy, 144
autoimmune diabetes, 6, 15–16
autoinjectors, 70
autonomic neuropathy, 124
Avandamet, 57, s59
Avandia, 58, 59, 170. *See also*
    thiazolidinediones (TZDs)
Aventis, 61

basal insulin, 27, 61, 63
Benson, Herbert, 144, 145
beta cells, 2, 6, 8, 17
    destruction of, by immune system,
        15, 16
    and exercise, 78
    exhaustion of, 5
    transplant of, 160
Bierman, June, 31–32, 147
biofeedback, 144–45
blood-glucose levels, 22–23, 25. *See*
    also blood-glucose testing
    and exercise, 77–78, 80
    high, 1, 5, 31
    monitoring, 74, 95–97, 109, 111
    Pattern Approach to managing, 35
    record keeping, 150, 152

blood-glucose levels, *continued*
and skin conditions, 87
and stress, 139, 140, 141
testing supplies and equipment for
monitoring, 104–9
and Type 1 diabetes, 25
blood-glucose meters, 106–9, 110, 166
blood-glucose testing, 34, 80, 97, 99
children and, 23
daily, 97, 100
earliest, 2
fasting and, 96, 97
frequency of, 96–97
insulin management methods and,
100–3
record keeping, 152
regular, 95
research on internal sensors,
163–64
supplies and equipment, 104–9
blood-glucose test strips, 106
blood-insulin levels
basal, 27
blood-sugar level and, 1, 5
blood pressure, 77
blood sugar. *See* blood-glucose levels
blood tests, 26, 34
board certified advanced diabetes
management (BC-ADM), 33, 37
body weight, ideal, 44
borderline diabetic, 6
Borg Scale of Perceived Exertion, 79
breathing
deep, 143
labored, 114
brittle diabetes, 141

calcium, 43
calories
adjusting for exercise, 80
requirements, 44–45
candidiasis, 87
capsaicin, 124
carbohydrates, 40, 41
counting, 45–46
cardiac monitor, 26
cardiomyopathy, 126
cardiovascular disease, 126,
128–29

Centers for Disease Control, 12
cerebral vascular disease (CVD), 129
certified diabetes educator (CDE),
33, 36
chemical diabetes, 13
children with diabetes
blood-glucose testing and, 23
caloric needs, 44–45
and exercise, 30
food and, 27
oral agents and, 54
parents of, 24, 136
renal thresholds and, 98
treatment of, 21–25
and Type 1 diabetes, 5
chlorpropamide, 54
cholesterol, 42
lowering, through exercise, 77
complementary health care choices,
158–59
complications of diabetes, 2–3,
11–12, 113–32. *See also*
Diabetes Control and
Complications Trial;
hypoglycemia; kidneys;
macroangiopathy; neuropathy;
retinopathy
acute, 114–18
chronic, 122–30
intermediate, 118–21
level of control of blood glucose,
23–24
managing, 35
continuous monitoring system
(CMS), 74
control of diabetes. *See also*
dietary control of diabetes;
self-management
aging and, 30
level of, and complications,
23–24
lifestyle and, 27
pregnancy and, 30-31
team management required for,
149–53
Type 1 diabetes, 26–29
Type 2 diabetes, 29–30
cortisol, 140
costs, national, of diabetes, 12

counselors, 134, 150
C-Peptide, 9
cranial mononeuropathy, 126

defense mechanisms, 135–36
depression, 135, 136
dental care, 85–86
designer insulins, 39
DiaBeta, 55, 56
Diabetes Care, 158
Diabetes Control and Complications
    Trial (DCCT), 23–24, 45, 130,
    170–72
Diabetes Forecast Resource Guide,
    104, 105
diabetes mellitus. *See also* Type 1
    diabetes mellitus; Type 2
    diabetes mellitus
  causes of, 15–17, 168–70
  classification of, 6, 7–8
  complications resulting from, 11
  cost of, 12
  defined, 1–2
  early forms of, 13
  facts and figures about, 18–19
  history of, 1–3
  increase in, 11–12, 18–19
  monitoring, 95–96
  problems associated with, 8–9
  research on cause and prevention,
      168–70
  treatment of, 2, 21–32
  types of, 1, 3–8, 13–15
Diabetes Prevention Program (DPP),
    169–70
Diabetes Prevention Trial (DPT), 169
Diabetes Self-Management, 109
Diabetes 2001 Vital Statistics, 11
Diabetes Type 2 Prevention
    Trial, 78
diabetic amyotrophy, 124
diabetic ketoacidosis (DKA), 3–4, 8,
    24, 114–15
  prediction of, 22
diabetic ketosis, 114
diabetogenic state, 30
diagnosis of diabetes
  criteria for, 5–6
  reaction to, 133–37

dietary control of diabetes, 39–50.
    See also food
  carbohydrate counting method,
      45–46
  eating guidelines, basic, 40–43
  high-protein diets, 48, 49–50
  meal planning, 39, 43–47
  point system methods, 46
  special needs and, 47–50
dietitian, 149–50
distal symmetrical polyneuro-
    pathy, 124
drugs. *See also* insulin; medications
    for diabetes
  as cause of diabetes, 14
Dymelor, 55

Edmonton Protocol, 160
education about diabetes, 12, 24, 26,
    33–38
  basic "survival" level, 33–34
  DCCT on, 170–71
  for family and friends, 137–38,
      156–57
  home-management level,
      34–35
  self-management levels, 35–36
education programs
  bringing family member or friend,
      156–57
  certification of, 33, 36, 37
  choosing, 36–37
  value of, 37–38
electrolytes, 114
Eli Lilly & Co., 61, 71
exchange system, 46
exercise
  benefits of, 77–80
  cholesterol and, 48
  for eyes, 91
  for feet, 89
  and managing diabetes, 30,
      77–78
  precautions in, 80–83
  prescription for, 83–84
  stress and, 145
exercise specialists, 150
eye care, 90–91. *See also* retinopathy
  and exercising, 83

family and friends
  and complementary and alternative
    choices in care, 158
  educating, 137–38, 155–56
  grieving by, 157
  support of, 137–38, 156–57
fasting plasma glucose level (FPG), 6
fats, 40, 41–42
feet. *See* foot care; shoes
fiber, dietary, 40
finger-stick test, 34
fluids, 22, 25, 49, 114–15
food. *See also* dietary control of
    diabetes
  absorption, 40
  adjusting intake of, 27, 44–45,
    47–48, 49, 82
  distribution throughout day, 40,
    44, 46
Food Guide Pyramid, 41
  stress and, 140–41
  Type 1 diabetes and, 27
foot care, 34, 87–90
friends. *See* family and friends
fructosamine test, 95, 99
funding for research, 172–73

General Adaptation Syndrome, 141
genetic factors. *See* heredity
gestational diabetes, 6, 13–14. *See
    also* pregnancy
gingivitis, 86
glargine (Lantus), 24, 28, 65–66,
    101, 121, 164–65
glimepiride (Amaryl), 55, 57, 59
glipizide (Glucotrol), 55, 56
glucagon, 2, 140
glucose. *See* blood-glucose levels
glucose toxicity, 5, 17
Glucophage, 57. *See also* metformins
Glucophage XR, 57. *See also*
    metformins
Glucotrol, 55, 56
Glucovance, 57, 59
GlucoWatch, 74, 164
glyburide (Micronase, Glynase), 55,
    56, 57, 59
glycosylated hemoglobin test, 95, 99

Glynase, 55, 56
Glyset, 57–58
grieving, 134–35, 157

healing touch, 147
health care costs, 12
health care team, 149–53
heart attacks, 129
heart rate, during exercise, 78–79
hemoglobin A1 test, 99
hemoglobin A1c, 99, 102, 111, 131
heparin lock, 26
heredity
  as cause of diabetes, 15, 16, 17
  research, 168–69
high-density lipoprotein (HDL),
    42, 77
HMOs, 109
home-management level of care,
    34–35
honeymoon period, 8, 27, 28
hormonal diseases, and secondary
    diabetes, 14
Humalog, 28, 29, 64, 66, 68, 71, 74,
    102, 121, 165
Human Regular insulin, 64, 65, 68,
    101, 102
Humulins, 65, 66, 71
hygiene, 34, 85
  dental care, 85–86
  eye care, 90–91
  foot care, 87–90
  in home management care, 34
  insulin delivery, 67
  sexually related, 91–93
  skin care, 86–87
hyperglycemia, 3, 23, 118
hyperglycemic hyperosmolar
    nonketotic syndrome, 14, 118
hypertension, 48
hypoglycemia, 22–23, 24, 48, 116–18

Idaho Plate Method, 45, 46–47
idiopathic diabetes, 6
Iletin II (R, N, L), 65
illness
  complications due to, 118–20
  and food intake, 49

imagery, 144
immune system
 and destruction of beta cells, 15, 16
 suppressing for transplants, 160
 Type 1 diabetes and, 15
immunosuppression, 160
impaired fasting glucose (IFG), 8, 13
impaired glucose homeostasis
 (IGH), 13
impaired glucose tolerance (IGT),
 8, 13
Insulflon, 72
insulin, 1, 2, 59–64. *See also* insulin
 injections; insulin management
 methods
 administering in children, 24
 animal derived, 59–60
 biologically engineered, 59
 delivery methods, 66–75
 designer, 39
 discovery of, 2
 doses, and carbohydrate
  counting, 45
 inhaled, 167
 intermediate-acting, 28, 65, 101
 lack of, in diabetes, 3, 4, 5, 6, 8
 long-acting, 65–66
 mixing, for injection, 67–68
 patterns of administration, 27–28
 premixed, 66
 rapid-acting, 28, 64–65, 101
 and relation to diabetes, 3, 4
 short-acting, 28, 65, 101
 side effects, 60
 types of, 28–29, 62–63, 64–66
insulin deficiency, 4, 5, 6, 17
insulin delivery methods,
 66–75
insulin injection, 68–74
 mixing insulin for injection, 67–68
 new methods, 166–67
 special instruments, 74–75
insulin-dependent diabetes mellitus.
 See Type 1 diabetes mellitus
insulin injections
 autoinjectors, 70
 blind persons and, 74–75
 improvements in, 166–67

insulin pumps, 72–74
jet injectors, 70–71
mixing insulins for, 67–68
multiple injection therapy, 72
needles and syringes, 69–70
pen injectors, 71
process of, 66–67, 68–69
insulin management methods,
 100–103
 algorithm approach, 100, 101–2
 patterned glucose approach, 35,
  102–3
 sliding scale methods, 101
 spacing throughout day, 102–3
insulin pumps, 72–74
insulin reactions, 22–23, 117
insulin resistance, 4, 17
intermittent claudication, 130
International Travel Association, 31
iron, 43
islets of Langerhans, 2, 15
 transplanting, 160, 161
isokinetic exercise, 79

Jackson, Robert L., 133
Juvenile Diabetes Foundation, 172
juvenile-onset diabetes. *See*
 Type 1 diabetes mellitus

ketoacidosis, diabetic. *See* diabetic
 ketoacidosis (DKA)
ketogenesis, 49, 118
ketones, 14
 defined, 3
 in diabetic ketoacidosis, 114,
  115, 118
 and exercising, 80
 in hyperglycemic hyperosmolar
  nonketotic syndrome, 118
 and Type 1 diabetes, 14
ketone tests, 22
ketosis, 114
kidneys
 damage to, 127
 transplant of, with pancreas, 161
Krieger, Delores, 147
Kuntz, Dora, 147
Kussmaul respiration, 114

lancets, 104–6
lancing devices, 105
Lantus, 64, 65–66, 68, 101, 102, 103, 121, 164–65
Lente, 28, 29, 60, 61, 64, 65, 68, 101, 102, 165
lifestyle
brittle diabetes and, 141
Type 1 diabetes and, 27
Type 2 diabetes and, 4
lispro (Humalog), 28, 29. *See also* Humalog
low-density lipoproteins (LDL), 42, 57, 77

macroangiopathy, 128–29
massage
gum, 86
therapeutic, 146
meal planning, 39, 43–47. *See also* dietary control of diabetes
medications for diabetes. *See also* insulin
insulin, 59–66
insulin delivery, 66–75
oral agents, 52–59
meditation, 144
meglitinides, 51, 54
Mentgen, Janet, 147
Metaglip, 59
meters, 106–9, 110
metformins (Glucophage, Glucophage XR), 52–53, 54, 57, 59
microangiopathy, 126–27
Micronase, 55, 56
miglitol (Glyset), 57–58
milk, and damage to beta cells, 16, 19
MODY (Maturity Onset Diabetes in the Young), 4. *See also* Type 2 diabetes mellitus
MUSE (medicated urethral system erection), 92

nasal inhalation of insulin, 167
nateglinide (Starlix), 55
National Diabetes Data Group, 11
National Institutes of Health, 172

nausea and vomiting, 34–35
necrobiosis lipoidica diabeticorum, 87
nephropathy, 127
Neurontin, 124
neuropathy, 122–26
non-insulin-dependent diabetes. *See* Type 2 diabetes mellitus
Novolins, 61, 65, 66, 71
Novolog, 28, 29, 64, 66, 68, 74, 102, 121, 165
Novo-Nordisk Pharmaceuticals, 61, 71
NPH (neutral protamine hagedorn), 28, 29, 61, 64, 65, 66, 68, 101, 102, 121, 165
numbness, 122, 123, 124
nurse educator, 149
nutrition, and stress, 145–46

obesity, and Type 2 diabetes, 4, 5. *See also* weight
ophthalmologists, 91
optometrists, 91–92
oral diabetes agents, 29–30, 52–59, 170
antihyperglycemic agents, 57–59
intermediate acting, 55–57
new, 170
short acting, 54–55
Orinase, 54

pancreas. *See also* beta cells
artificial, research on, 162–64
and idiopathic diabetes, 6
and milk protein, 19
pig, 162
and secondary diabetes, 3, 14
transplants, 159, 160–62
pancreatitis, 14
PARENT approach to stress management, 142–47
parents of children with diabetes, 24, 136. *See also* family and friends
Pattern Approach, to blood-glucose management, 35, 102–3
pen injectors, 71
peripheral vascular disease (PVD), 130

physicians
blood-glucose testing by, 96–97
knowledgeable, finding, 153
research funds and, 172–73
specialists, 150
pig
pancreas from, 162
insulin derived from, 59–60, 65
pink eye, 90
pioglitazone (Actos), 58, 59
plasma expanders, 114
podiatrists, 89, 150
point system, for dietary control, 46
polydipsia, 4
polyphagia, 4, 5
polyuria, 3, 4
pork insulin, 59–60, 65
positive thinking, 142
potassium, 114, 115, 118
Prandin, 54–55
Precose, 57–58
prediabetes, 13, 129
pregnancy
complications with, 120–21
development of diabetes and,
13–14
management of diabetes and,
30–31
renal thresholds and, 98
progressive relaxation, 143
prostaglandin, 92
protamine, 60
proteins, 40, 42–43
liquid high-protein diets, 48, 49–50
proximal motor neuropathy, 124, 126
psychologists, 134, 150

quality of life, 22

radiculopathy, 126
"rainbow therapy," 100
Reavens, George, 129
record keeping, 150–53
Regular insulin. *See* Human Regular
insulin
relaxation techniques, 142–45
remission, partial, Type 1 diabetes, 8
renal threshold, 98–99
repaglinide (Prandin), 54–55

research
on cause and prevention, 168–70
funding for, 172–73
on implantable sensors, 163–64
on new treatments, 164–68
on transplants, 159–62
retinologists, 91
retinopathy, 2, 11, 128. *See also*
eye care
reverse iontophoresis, 164
rosiglitazone (Avandia), 57, 58, 59

salt intake, 48
Satcher, David, 12
secondary diabetes, 3, 14
self-esteem, 136–37
self-management, 33–36. *See also*
control of diabetes
DCCT on, 170–71
program management, 149–50
record keeping, 150–53
stress management, 142–47
support of family and friends,
137–38
self-monitoring of blood-glucose
(SMBG), 100, 109, 111
Self-Recognition, 36
Selye, Hans, 141
Semilente, 65
sexual functioning, 91–93
shoes, 89
skin
care of, 86–87
insulin delivery and preventing
infection in, 69, 74
sliding scale method of insulin
management, 101
snacks, 48, 80
social workers, 150
sodium chloride, 48, 114
Starlix, 55
sticks (blood-glucose test strips), 106
stress
acute response to, 139–40
chronic response to, 140–41
complications due to, 118–20
managing, 142–47
pregnancy and, 30–31
Type 1 diabetes and, 3

SugarFree Centers, 31
sugar toxicity, 5, 17
sulfonylureas, 51, 55
support, of family members and
    friends, 137–38, 155–58
surgery, complications due to, 120
Sutherland, Donald, 161
syndrome X, 129

target zone, 78–79
T-cells, 16
team management of diabetes, 149–53
Tegretol, 124
therapeutic touch, 147
thiazolidinediones (TZDs), 51, 52,
    53, 58–59, 170
toenails, 88–89
tolazamide (Tolinase), 55, 56
tolbutamide (Orinase), 54
Tolinase, 55
Toohey, Barbara, 31, 147
touch, 146–47
transplants, 159–62
    artificial pancreas transplants,
        162–64
travel
    and complications during, 121
    and managing diabetes, 31–32
treatment of diabetes, 21–32
    acute care, 25–26
    children versus adults, 21–25
    managing Type 1 diabetes, 26–29
    managing Type 2 diabetes, 29–30
    special management needs, 30–32
triglycerides, 42, 77
Type 1 diabetes mellitus, 3, 5
    acute care of, 25–26
    causes of, 15–17
    defined, 3, 5
    and exercise, 82
    and eye exams, 91
    heredity and, 168–69
    increase in, 18
    insulin deficiency an, 6
    lifestyle and, 27
    management of, 26–29, 170–72
    problems of, 8
    subclasses of, 6
    symptoms of, 14–15

various names for, 14
versus Type 2, 4–5
Type 2 diabetes mellitus, 4, 5–6
    causes of, 17–18
    defined, 4
    and exercise, 30
    and eye exams, 91
    heredity and, 168
    increase in, 18
    lifestyle and, 4
    management of, 29–30, 170–72
    new therapies for, 167–68
    oral medication for, 51–59
    problems of, 9
    research on prevention of, 169–70
    subclasses of, 6
    various names for, 4
    versus Type 1, 4–5

Ultralente, 28, 60, 64, 65, 101, 121,
    165
unconsciousness, 116, 129
United Kingdom Prospective Diabetes
    Study (UKPDS), 131, 171, 172
urine tests, 98–99, 104, 131

Velosolin, 66, 74
very low density lipoproteins
    (VLDL), 129
Viagra, 92
visually impaired persons, 74–75.
    See also eye care; retinopathy
vitamin supplements, 43, 48

walking, 89
weight. See also obesity
    calculating ideal, 44
    losing, 47–48
women and diabetes. See gestational
    diabetes; pregnancy
World Health Organization, 11

xanthoma, 87

yeast infections, 87

Z-tracking, 69